ADVANCES IN SURGICAL PATHOLOGY

MESOTHELIOMA

ADVANCES IN SURGICAL PATHOLOGY SERIES

SERIES EDITORS: **Philip T. Cagle, MD, and Timothy C. Allen, MD, JD**

Advances in Surgical Pathology: Lung Cancer
Philip T. Cagle and Timothy C. Allen, *2010*

Advances in Surgical Pathology: Gastric Cancer
Dongfeng Tan and Gregory Y. Lauwers, *2010*

Advances in Surgical Pathology: Endometrial Cancer
Anna Sienko, *2012*

Advances in Surgical Pathology: Prostate Cancer
Jae Y. Ro, Steven S. Shen, and Alberto G. Ayala, *2012*

Advances in Surgical Pathology: Mesothelioma
Richard L. Attanoos and Timothy Craig Allen, *2013*

Advances in Surgical Pathology: Colorectal Carcinoma and Tumors of the Vermiform Appendix
Rhonda K. Yantiss, *2013*

Advances in Surgical Pathology: Breast Cancer
Omar Hameed, Mohamed Mokhtar Desouki, Heidi R. Umphrey, and Shi Wei, *2014*

Advances in Surgical Pathology: Thyroid Cancer
Mojgan Amrikachi and Rose Anton, *2015*

Advances in Surgical Pathology: Brain Cancer
Andreana Rivera and Hidehiro Takei, *2015*

ADVANCES IN SURGICAL PATHOLOGY

MESOTHELIOMA

Richard L. Attanoos, MBBS, FRCPath

Consultant Pathologist
Department of Pathology
University Hospital Llandough
APC (Pathology) Ltd
Cardiff, Wales, United Kingdom

Timothy Craig Allen, MD, JD

Professor of Pathology
Chairman, Department of Pathology
The University of Texas Health Science Center at Tyler
Tyler, Texas

SERIES EDITORS

Philip T. Cagle, MD

Professor of Pathology and Laboratory Medicine
Weill Medical College of Cornell University
New York, New York
Director, Pulmonary Pathology
The Methodist Hospital
Houston, Texas

Timothy Craig Allen, MD, JD

Professor of Pathology
Chairman, Department of Pathology
The University of Texas Health Science Center
at Tyler
Tyler, Texas

Wolters Kluwer | Lippincott Williams & Wilkins
Health

Philadelphia • Baltimore • New York • London
Buenos Aires • Hong Kong • Sydney • Tokyo

Acquisitions Editor: Ryan Shaw
Product Manager: Kate Marshall
Production Project Manager: David Orzechowski
Senior Manufacturing Coordinator: Beth Welsh
Marketing Manager: Alexander Burns
Designer: Stephen Druding
Production Service: SPi Global

Two Commerce Square
2001 Market Street
Philadelphia, PA 19103 USA
LWW.com

Printed in China

Library of Congress Cataloging-in-Publication Data
Attanoos, Richard L.
Advances in surgical pathology. Mesothelioma / Richard L. Attanoos, Timothy Craig Allen. — 1st ed.
p. ; cm. — (Advances in surgical pathology series)
Mesothelioma
Includes bibliographical references and index.
ISBN 978-1-60831-618-2 (hardback)
I. Allen, Timothy C. II. Title. III. Title: Mesothelioma. IV. Series: Advances in surgical pathology series.
[DNLM: 1. Mesothelioma—pathology. 2. Mesothelioma—diagnosis. QZ 340]
RC280.L8
616.99'424—dc23

2013014767

---

10 9 8 7 6 5 4 3 2 1

RRS1306

Series Overview

Expectations for the pathologist practicing today exceed those for pathologists in practice only a few years ago. In addition to the rapid growth of knowledge and new technologies in the field of pathology, recent years have seen the emergence of many trends that significantly impact the traditional practice of pathology including the subspecialized multidisciplinary approach to patient care; personalized therapeutics including targeted molecular therapies; and imaging techniques such as endoscopic microscopy, molecular radiology, and imaging multimodality theranostics that compete with conventional light microscopy. In order to remain a viable member of the patient care team, the pathologist must keep up with growing knowledge in traditional subjects as well as in new areas of expertise such as molecular testing. Additionally, the pathologist is subject to an increasing number of credentialing requirements and, for those now completing training, Self-Assessment Modules for Maintenance of Certification, which require the pathologist to be examined on the recent advances in pathology in order to sustain their qualifications to practice.

Each volume in the new series *Advances in Surgical Pathology* focuses on a specific subject in pathology that has undergone recent advancement in terms of knowledge, technical procedures, application and/or integration as part of current trends in pathology and medicine. This series of books not only updates the pathologist on recently acquired knowledge but emphasizes the new uses of that knowledge within the context of the changing landscape of pathology practice in the 21st century. Rather than information in a vacuum, the pathologist is educated on how to apply the new knowledge as part of a subspecialized multidisciplinary team and for purposes of personalized patient therapy.

Each volume in the series will be divided into following sections: (1) Overview—Updates the pathologist on the general topic, including epidemiology, bringing the pathologist generally up-to-date on a topic as a basis for the more specialized sections that follow. (2) Histopathology—Reviews histopathology and specific recent changes that warrant more description and more illustration, for example, recently described entities and recent revisions in classifications. This will also emphasize histopathology figures to illustrate recently described entities and to demonstrate the basis for classification changes so that the pathologist is able to understand and recognize these changes. (3) Imaging—Reviews the impact of imaging techniques on histopathologic diagnosis and on the practice of pathology. An example of the former is the use of increasingly sensitive high-resolution computed tomography scan in the diagnosis of interstitial lung diseases. An example of the latter is the use of multimodality theranostics rather than traditional histopathology for the diagnosis and treatment of lung cancer. Figures linking the radiologic images to the histopathology will be emphasized. (4) Molecular Pathology—A review and update on specific molecular pathology as it applies to specific diseases for the practicing pathologist in regards to molecular diagnostics and molecular therapeutics. An example of the former is the identification of a specific fusion gene to diagnose synovial sarcoma. An example of the latter is the identification of specific epidermal growth factor receptor (EGFR) mutations in pulmonary adenocarcinoma and its relationship to treatment with EGFR antagonists. (5) For those volumes dealing with cancers (Lung Cancer, Breast Cancer, Prostate Cancer, Colon Cancer, etc.), additional sections will include Preneoplastic and Preinvasive Lesions, which will emphasize histopathologic figures and staging, particularly emphasizing the new staging systems and to illustrate specific problems in staging.

These books will assist the pathologist in daily practice in the modern setting and provide a basis for interacting with other physicians in patient care. They will also provide the timely updates in knowledge that is necessary for daily practice, for current credentialing, and for Maintenance of Certification. As such, this series is invaluable to pathologists in practice at all levels of experience who need to keep up with advances for their daily performance and their periodic credentialing and to pathologists-in-training who will apply this knowledge to their boards and their future practice. In the latter case, this series will serve as a useful library for pathology training programs.

To Emma, Josef, and Lily
—Richard L. Attanoos

To my children Erin and Caitlin,
and to my wife Fran
—Timothy Craig Allen

Contributors

Timothy Craig Allen, MD, JD
Professor of Pathology
Chairman, Department of Pathology
The University of Texas Health Science Center at Tyler
Tyler, Texas

Richard L. Attanoos, MBBS, FRCPath
Consultant Pathologist
Department of Pathology
University Hospital Llandough
APC (Pathology) Ltd
Cardiff, Wales, United Kingdom

Alain C. Borczuk, MD
Professor of Clinical Pathology
Columbia University Medical Center
New York, New York

Allen R. Gibbs, MBChB, FRCPath
Consultant Pathologist
Department of Cellular Pathology
University Hospital Llandough
Penarth, United Kingdom

Jason Lester, MRCP, FRCR
Consultant Oncologist
Velindre Cancer Centre
Cardiff, Wales, United Kingdom

Preface

Diffuse malignant mesothelioma is rare. There are many times more primary and metastatic neoplasms that involve the serosal surfaces that mimic diffuse malignant mesothelioma than there are actual diffuse malignant mesotheliomas. Moreover, diffuse malignant mesothelioma's wide variety of histologic appearances are mimicked not only by other primary and metastatic neoplasms, but also very common reactive conditions involving the serosal surfaces can be so histologically robust as to mimic diffuse malignant mesothelioma as well. The diagnosis of diffuse malignant mesothelioma is therefore frequently far from straightforward.

In addition, given the dismal outcome of almost all patients with diffuse malignant mesothelioma, as well as the dearth of successful therapeutic options, the diagnosis of diffuse malignant mesothelioma, once rendered, carries with it enormous prognostic weight. Legal considerations add another level of complexity, and they often arise as soon as the diagnosis of diffuse malignant mesothelioma is clinically considered, much less pathologically rendered. Unfortunately, these legal considerations may intentionally or unintentionally influence, or attempt to influence, the pathologist examining the case.

Even as the incidence and mortality of diffuse malignant mesothelioma are expected to increase, desperately needed molecular-based therapies that have shown benefit in patients with cancers such as breast and lung have yet to provide any therapeutic benefit in patients with diffuse malignant mesothelioma. Nonetheless, researchers are carefully studying the molecular mechanisms involved in asbestos-caused diffuse malignant mesothelioma in an attempt to identify molecular diagnostic, prognostic, and therapeutic biomarkers for which new, promising therapies may be based.

Also, besides diffuse malignant mesothelioma, there are other, even rarer, mesotheliomas which have not been shown to be caused by asbestos exposure, and which have differing prognoses and treatments. It is imperative that these be accurately diagnosed as well.

This book is meant to address the diagnostic aspects of mesothelioma as well as the ongoing molecular research surrounding diffuse malignant mesothelioma. It is meant to assist the pathologist in diagnosing diffuse malignant mesothelioma and other mesotheliomas, as well as to differentiate the much more common lesions that mimic diffuse malignant mesothelioma, with particular attention to reactive mesothelial hyperplasia and fibrous pleuritis.

The editors wish to gratefully acknowledge our esteemed predecessors and colleagues whose expertise in mesothelioma has added much to our understanding of this devastating disease.

Richard L. Attanoos, MBBS, FRCPath
Timothy Craig Allen, MD, JD

Contents

ADVANCES IN SURGICAL PATHOLOGY

MESOTHELIOMA

SECTION

I

Epidemiologic, Clinical, and Radiologic Features

1 The Diagnosis of Mesothelioma

▶ Timothy Craig Allen
▶ Richard L. Attanoos

The diagnosis of mesothelioma is one of the most difficult diagnostic challenges a pathologist may ever face. Mesothelioma is an extremely uncommon diagnosis, and some pathologists remain unfamiliar with its diagnosis for their entire careers. It is also a neoplasm that exhibits a wide variety of histologic patterns, for which there are a correspondingly large number of mimics, both neoplastic and nonneoplastic. The remoteness of the diagnosis of asbestos-related mesothelioma from the patient's initial asbestos exposure, often occurring decades before, may make diagnosis more difficult. Further, the diagnosis of diffuse malignant mesothelioma carries with it a dismal prognosis, making misdiagnosis a potentially serious misadventure. Finally, its diagnosis—indeed, its mere suggestion—almost invariably ignites legal overtures.

The starkly dismal prognosis of diffuse malignant mesothelioma is well known. Few patients survive more than 2 years; most do not survive even 1 year after diagnosis. Conventional treatments—surgical, chemotherapeutic, and radiotherapeutic—are of limited benefit, at best providing only a few months of survival benefit. And while recent molecular diagnostic and therapeutic discoveries have altered, and even revolutionized, diagnosis and treatment of other cancers, such as breast cancer and lung cancer, patients with diffuse malignant mesothelioma have not yet benefited from the expansion of molecular medicine.

Although very few long-term survivors of diffuse malignant mesothelioma have been identified by expert pulmonary pathologists, such as those in the International Mesothelioma Panel, almost all cases of "long-term survival" of diffuse malignant mesothelioma represent misdiagnoses. For reasons of diagnostic accuracy, therapeutic appropriateness, legal certainty, and research integrity, accurate diagnosis of diffuse malignant mesothelioma is vital. This book is meant to reinforce, educate, and clarify important issues surrounding the diagnosis of diffuse malignant mesothelioma, as well as other mesotheliomas, and to explain current and ongoing features surrounding the molecular basis of diffuse malignant mesothelioma.

WHO Classification

2

Richard L. Attanoos

The serosal tissues are site to a wide spectrum of tumors and tumor-like conditions. The most important is diffuse malignant mesothelioma, which represents the most significant occupational cancer worldwide because of its association with asbestos. There exist many unresolved controversies regarding the relationship between diffuse malignant mesothelioma and asbestos.

Primary tumors of the serosa have been classified dependent on anatomic site (pleura versus peritoneum), and there exists no ideal classification system. The nomenclature of many of these conditions has evolved over recent years; some counterpart lesions have been recognized in different serosal sites, but notable differences remain, which precludes against a comfortable emergence of a universally agreed classification system for tumors of the serosa. Serosal tumors may be classified according to their likely histogenetic cell of origin: mesothelial, submesothelial mesenchymal, and uncertain (uncommitted stem cells). In each compartment, there are reported tumors whose biologic behavior ranges from benign to malignant. The World Health Organization formulated a classification of tumors of the pleura[1] and peritoneum.[2]

WHO HISTOLOGIC CLASSIFICATION OF SEROSAL TUMORS: SITE-SPECIFIC DIFFERENCES

Mesothelial Tumors

Diffuse Malignant Mesothelioma

Diffuse malignant mesothelioma is the most common primary malignant neoplasm arising from the serosa. Most cases occur in the pleura with approximately 10% to 20% arising in the peritoneum and approximately 1% in the tunica vaginalis testis, ovary, and pericardium. The 2004 World Health Organization classification of lung and pleural tumors recognizes four major histologic subtypes of diffuse malignant mesothelioma: epithelioid, biphasic, sarcomatoid, and desmoplastic (Figs. 2-1 to 2-4). The epithelioid and sarcomatoid subtypes may occur in pure form or in a morphologic combination in biphasic (mixed) subtype tumor. Cytologic and nuclear atypia and mitotic activity vary from mild to marked in the different variant forms. The most common morphologic pattern of diffuse malignant mesothelioma at all serosal sites is pure epithelioid subtype with tubulopapillary elements; however, the histologic appearance of diffuse malignant mesothelioma is quite protean, with a diversity of histologic variants identified.

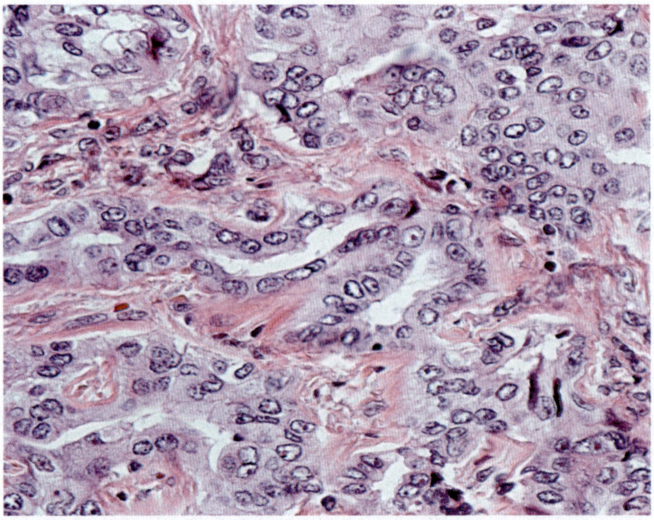

FIGURE 2-1: Epithelioid diffuse malignant mesothelioma, with tubular structures that may mimic adenocarcinoma.

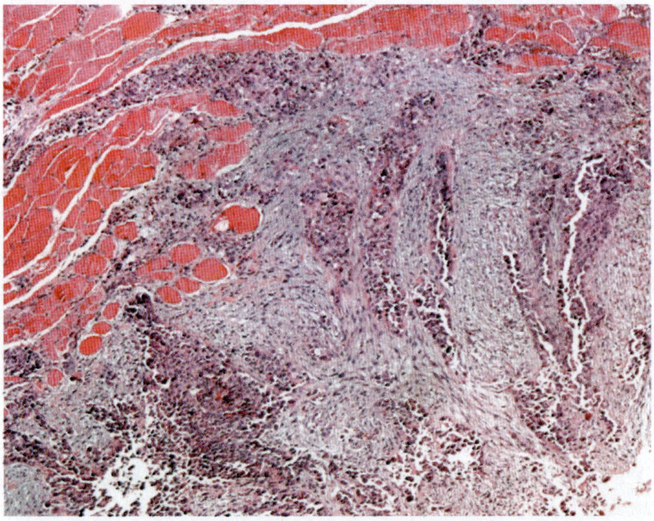

FIGURE 2-2: Biphasic diffuse malignant mesothelioma, containing both epithelioid and sarcomatoid components, invading skeletal muscle.

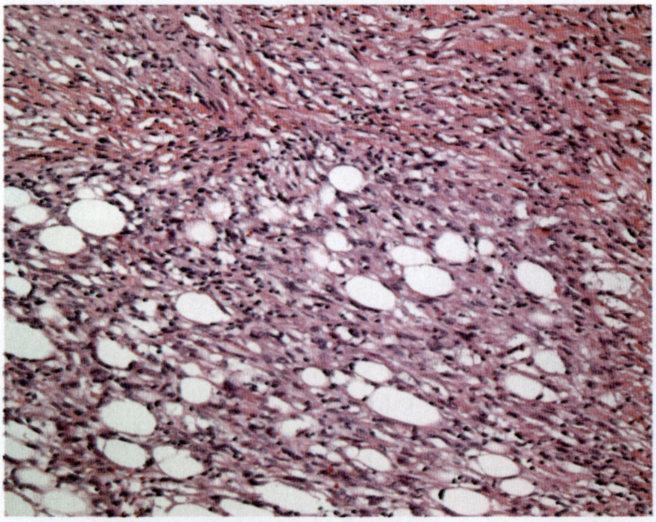

FIGURE 2-3: Sarcomatoid diffuse malignant mesothelioma invading chest wall adipose tissue.

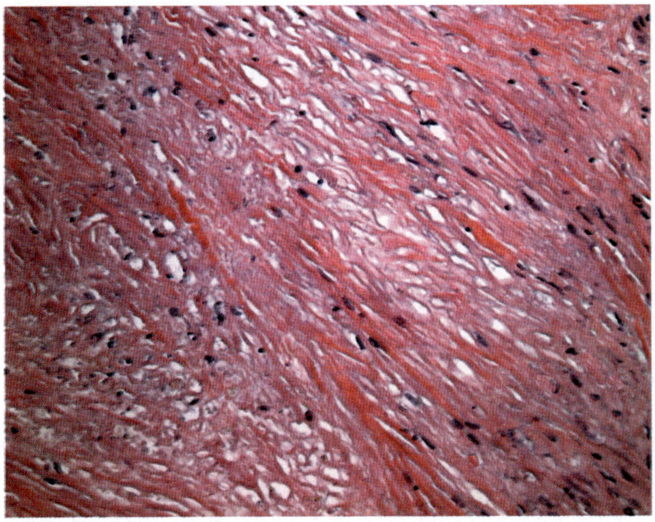

FIGURE 2-4: Desmoplastic diffuse malignant mesothelioma with scant cellularity in a dense fibrous background.

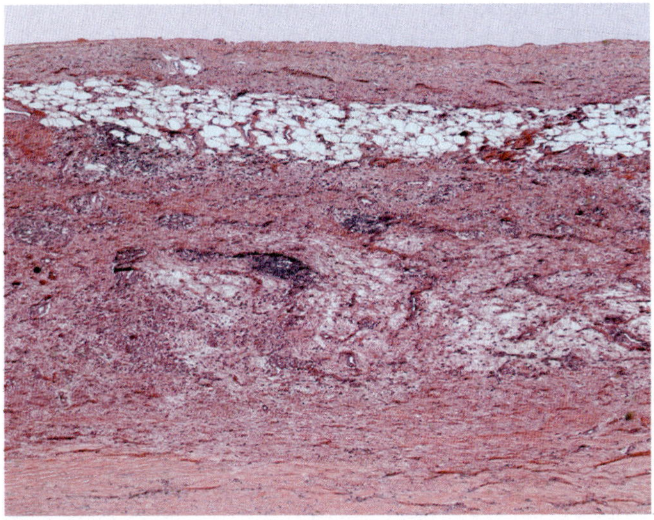

FIGURE 2-5: Fibrous pleuritis, which may mimic sarcomatoid diffuse malignant mesothelioma.

The recognition of desmoplastic diffuse malignant mesothelioma as a separate histologic subtype is controversial. It is most likely a variant of sarcomatoid subtype diffuse malignant mesothelioma. The diagnosis of desmoplastic diffuse malignant mesothelioma requires there be a predominant (>50%) component of dense collagenous stroma containing paucicellular and haphazardly arranged atypical nucleated cells. Most desmoplastic diffuse malignant mesotheliomas contain areas of otherwise typical sarcomatoid diffuse malignant mesothelioma. Rarely, the minority tumor component is biphasic or epithelioid subtype tumor. Most desmoplastic diffuse malignant mesotheliomas are reported in the pleura; primary peritoneal diffuse malignant mesothelioma of desmoplastic subtype is exceptionally rare. Currently, desmoplastic tumors are generally considered to be a subclassification of sarcomatoid diffuse malignant mesotheliomas; the only reasons for considering desmoplastic diffuse malignant mesothelioma as an independent, distinct, subtype are its particularly poor prognosis and the ease at which it can be misinterpreted as chronic fibrosing pleurisy (Fig. 2-5)—not sufficient for its retention of individual subclassification status.

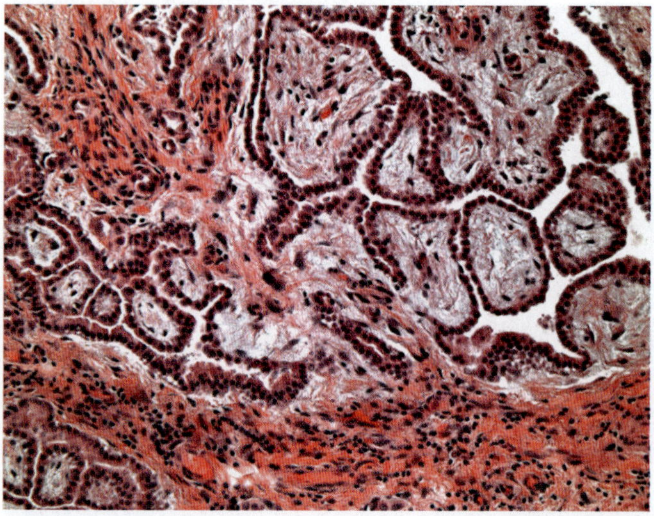

FIGURE 2-6: Well-differentiated papillary mesothelioma.

Most peritoneal diffuse malignant mesotheliomas are epithelioid subtype tumors, with pure sarcomatoid subtype tumors appearing far less commonly in the peritoneum than in the pleura. This may represent a true site-specific variation or, because primary peritoneal mesotheliomas are far less amenable to radical surgery than pleural tumors, reflect sampling error.

Well-Differentiated Papillary Mesothelioma

Well-differentiated papillary mesothelioma is far more common in the female pelvic peritoneum, although rare cases in the pleura have been identified (Fig. 2-6). The tumor is important to recognize and distinguish from diffuse malignant mesothelioma, because well-differentiated papillary mesothelioma has no recognized association with asbestos. It must be emphasized that there is no recognized counterpart "poorly differentiated" papillary mesothelioma, which can be readily defined and distinguished from diffuse malignant mesothelioma.

Cystic Mesothelioma

Cystic mesothelioma, also termed multicystic mesothelioma, is recognized in the WHO Classification of the peritoneum (2003) but not in the 2004 classification of pleural tumors (Fig. 2-7). The vast majority of cystic mesotheliomas are reported in the female peritoneum but pleural counterpart lesions exist. It is controversial whether these are truly neoplastic or are post inflammatory tumor-like lesions.

Adenomatoid Tumor

Adenomatoid tumor, previously ambiguously termed "benign mesothelioma," is usually reported in the pleura or in association with genital tract organs (Fig. 2-8). Strict diagnostic criteria must be adhered to. Adenomatoid tumors are typically small, occult findings with characteristic morphology. Rare combinations of adenomatoid tumor, cystic mesothelioma, and well-differentiated papillary mesothelioma have been reported in the peritoneum, which points to a possible similar etiologic origin, as all of these are unrelated to asbestos.

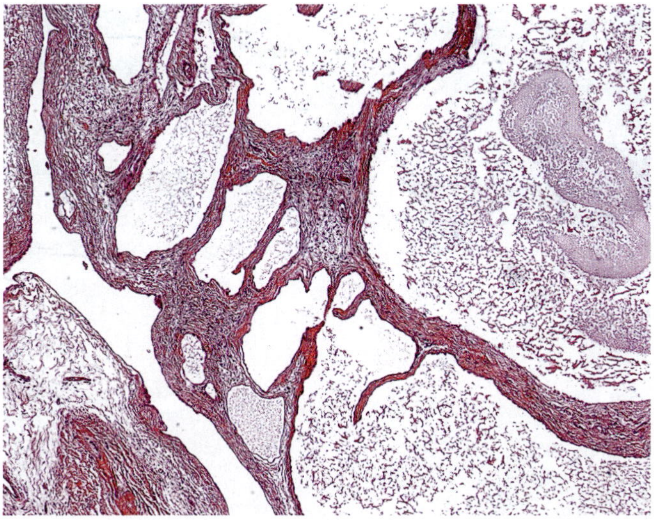

FIGURE 2-7: Cystic mesothelioma.

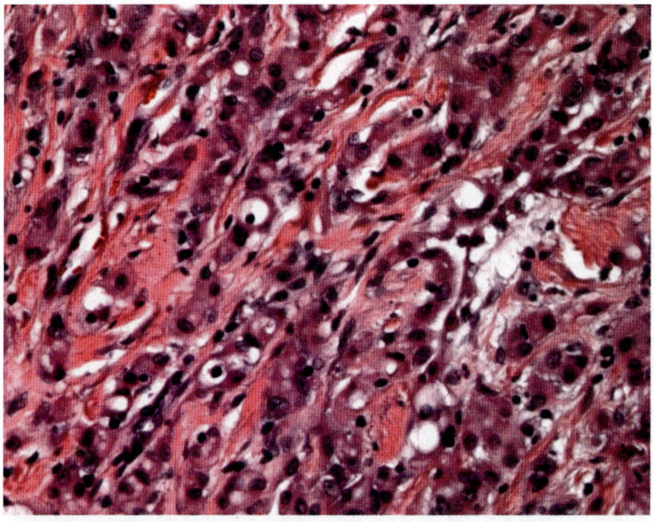

FIGURE 2-8: Adenomatoid tumor.

Submesothelial Mesenchymal Tumors

The submesothelial tissues exhibit a diverse plasticity with the potential to undergo epithelioid and mesenchymal spindle cell differentiation. A wide variety of mesenchymal tumors have been reported in pleural, peritoneal, and pericardial sites. Solitary fibrous tumors (benign and malignant counterparts), (epithelioid) vascular sarcomas, and synovial sarcomas are well reported. Calcifying fibrous tumor, inflammatory myofibroblastic tumor, and desmoid tumor (fibromatosis) reported at varied serosal sites are not consistently represented in existing classification systems (Figs. 2-9 and 2-10). This may well reflect the continuing uncertainty of the histogenesis or nature of the individual lesions. The so-called omental mesenteric myxoid hamartoma is likely synonymous with some forms of inflammatory myofibroblastic tumor with distinct clinicopathologic features.

Childhood serosal tumors are primitive thoracopulmonary neuroectodermal tumors (Askin tumor); pleuropulmonary blastoma is rare and has been reported in the pleura. Desmoplastic small round cell tumor is recognized in both 2004 pleural and 2003 peritoneal classifications reported in the abdominal, pelvic, pleural, and paratesticular regions (Fig. 2-11).

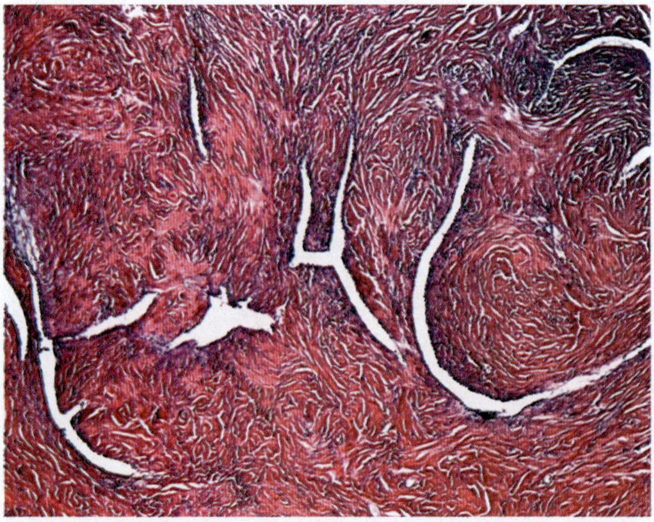

FIGURE 2-9: Solitary fibrous tumor of the pleura.

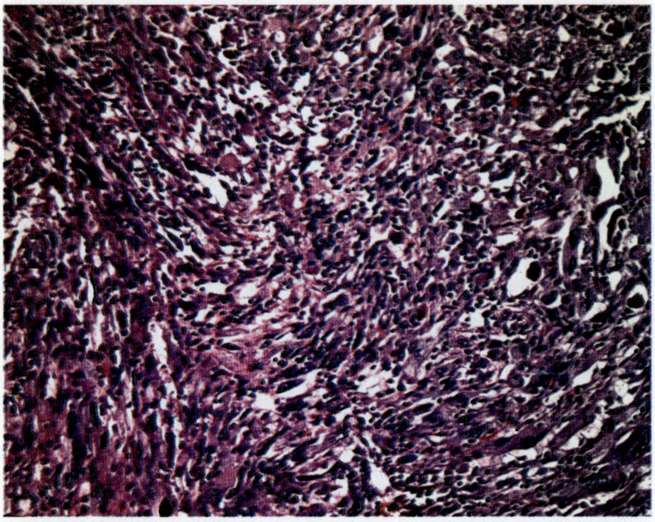

FIGURE 2-10: Malignant solitary fibrous tumor of the pleura, showing increased cellularity.

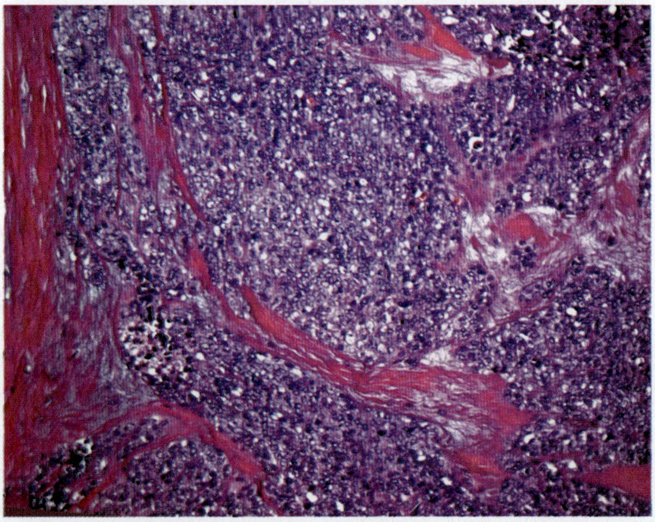

FIGURE 2-11: Desmoplastic small round cell tumor.

In the peritoneum, there exist a variety of conditions of likely metaplastic origin exhibiting end differentiation of subserosal mesenchymal cells—such as leiomyomatosis peritonealis disseminata, gliomatosis peritonei, omental deciduosis, and osseous and chondroid metaplasia. Because the processes are of metaplastic origin, it is contentious to include them in a tumor classification system. Nonetheless, leiomyomatosis peritonealis disseminata is well recognized as a potential pitfall of metastatic malignancy in the peritoneum and associated with leiomyomas, endometriosis, pregnancy, and oral contraceptive use.

PRIMARY EPITHELIAL TUMORS OF THE PERITONEUM

Embryologic studies show that the peritoneum and the Mullerian duct derivatives share a common coelomic epithelial ancestry. In the female pelvic peritoneum, primary epithelial lesions exist, which resemble either the normal epithelial elements of the female reproductive organs or their neoplastic counterparts.

The literature contains a wide spectrum of primary peritoneal Mullerian tumors. The most recognized tumors are primary peritoneal serous carcinoma and serous borderline tumor. These are identical to their ovarian counterparts. The majority of serous carcinomas are high grade and have a complex, variably papillary, glandular, and solid architecture, with marked cytologic atypia and mitotic activity. Psammoma bodies are frequently present. Their behavior is similar to or worse than that of stage III ovarian serous carcinoma.

Serous borderline tumors of the peritoneum are identical to serous borderline ovarian tumors. The diagnosis of a primary peritoneal serous borderline tumor can only be made in

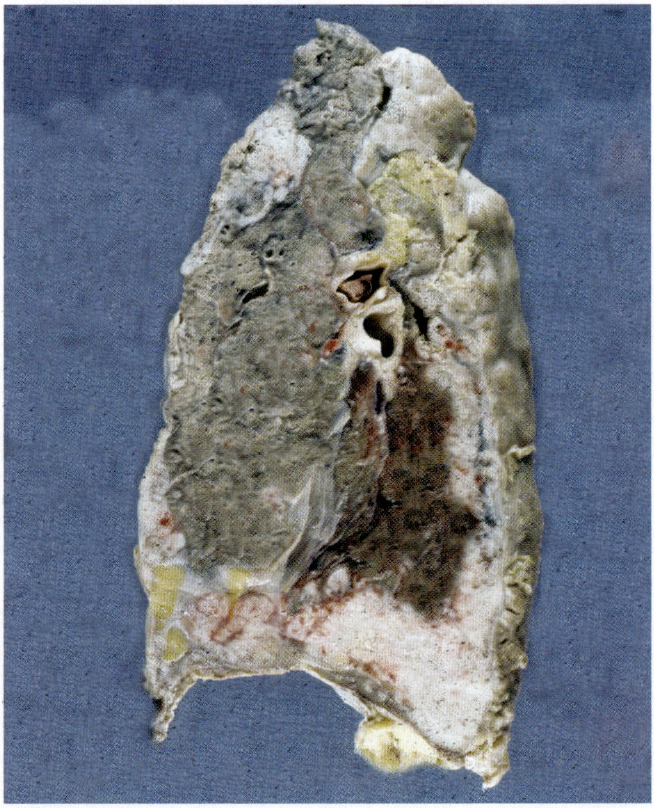

FIGURE 2-12: Gross image of pseudomesotheliomatous adenocarcinoma of the lung, showing the rind-like pattern of tumor spread characteristic of diffuse malignant mesothelioma.

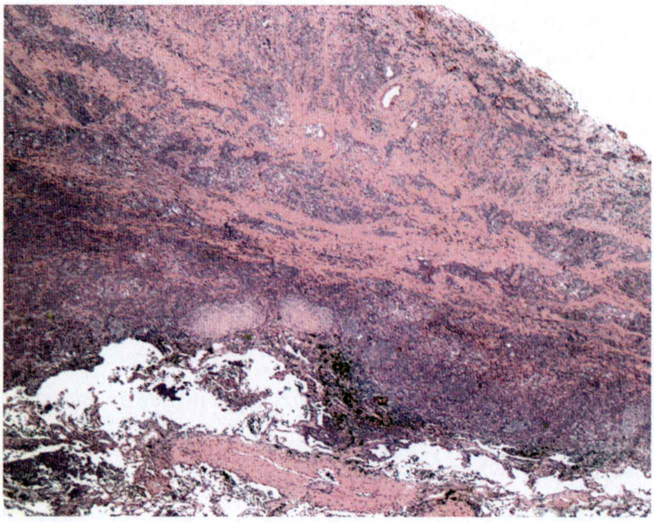

FIGURE 2-13: Pseudomesotheliomatous adenocarcinoma of the lung, showing pleural and subpleural tumor mimicking diffuse malignant mesothelioma.

the absence of ovarian involvement or when there is minimal surface involvement. Primary peritoneal serous borderline tumors show cellular stratification and tufting, detachment of cell groups, mild to moderate cytologic atypia, and mitotic activity, but there is no evidence of stromal invasion. These tumors may arise from foci of endosalpingiosis, which are present in most cases. These patients generally have a good prognosis, which is similar to that of patients with a serous borderline ovarian tumors and noninvasive peritoneal implants.

In the pleura, no counterpart primary epithelial tumor is recognized. By contrast, there exist a variety of so-called pseudomesotheliomatous tumors, most of which represent direct and diffuse involvement of the serosa by primary peripheral lung adenocarcinomas (Figs. 2-12 and 2-13).

References

1. Travis WD, Brambilla E, Muller-Hermelink HW, et al. *Pathology and Genetics of Tumors of the Lungs, Pleura, Mediastinum and Heart.* Lyon, France: WHO IARC; 2004.
2. Tavassoli FA, Devilee P. *Pathology and Genetics of Tumours of the Breast and Female Genital Organs.* Lyon, France: WHO IARC; 2003.

3 Staging

Jason Lester

Historically, the lack of a consensus staging system for diffuse malignant mesothelioma has had a detrimental effect on both clinical practice and research.[1] Comparing results between studies and centers was very difficult and hindered the medical management of patients with pleural diffuse malignant mesothelioma. The first formal staging system for pleural diffuse malignant mesothelioma that came to be widely adopted was by Butchart et al.,[2] which defined four stages of disease. The Butchart staging system was based on only 29 patients who had undergone extrapleural pneumonectomy. The Butchart staging system has been found to be significantly associated with survival in some series but unrelated in others.[3,4] The Butchart system was developed before the introduction of computed tomography (CT) scanning, so preoperative assessment was limited. Because virtually all patients who can be pathologically staged are classified as stage I or II, the prognostic utility of the system is limited.

Several subsequent modifications to the Butchart system were proposed over the next 20 years, most of which had limitations analogous to those of the Butchart system, and none was universally accepted and applied.[5,6] In 1997, the International Mesothelioma Interest Group (IMIG) was formed. The IMIG approved a staging system previously developed by some of the group's members with the objective of universal acceptance and implementation.[7] This staging system was accepted by the American Joint Committee on Cancer (AJCC) and the International Union against Cancer (UICC) and is published in their sixth and seventh editions, respectively.[8,9]

The UICC/AJCC staging system reflects the potential resectability of the disease. T1a tumors involve only the parietal pleura, and a complete macroscopic resection may be achieved with pleurectomy–decortication. With tumor growth into the visceral pleura (T1b/T2), the tumor cannot usually be removed by pleurectomy–decortication, necessitating extrapleural pneumonectomy. T3 describes a locally advanced tumor, but one that technically still may be resectable by extrapleural pneumonectomy. T4 tumors show extensive local advancement and are unresectable (Figs. 3-1 to 3-3).

The lymphatic drainage of the pleura is complex. Pleural diffuse malignant mesothelioma arises primarily from the parietal and diaphragmatic pleura, and therefore, extrapleural N2 nodes rather than intrapleural N1 nodes might be the first draining station. This makes interpretation of stage groupings difficult. The current pleural diffuse malignant mesothelioma staging system combines N1 and N2 disease as stage III because it is uncertain whether there is any prognostic difference between them. Surgical series in the literature are conflicting; Sugarbaker et al.[10] reported significantly shorter survival in those with N2 disease compared to those without. Allen et al.[11] reported no difference between the two groups. As more data become available, the impact of nodal status on prognosis will become clearer, and revisions of the UICC/AJCC staging system may be needed.

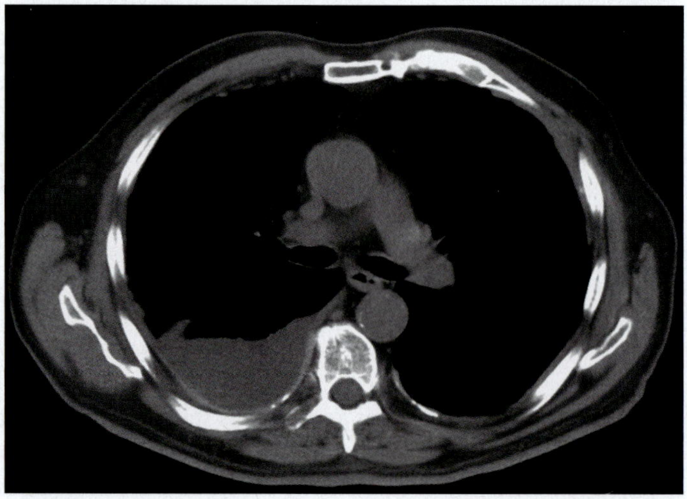

FIGURE 3-1: T1 disease. Axial CT scan showing minimal pleural thickening in the right hemithorax posteriorly. Note associated moderate right effusion, which does not influence disease stage.

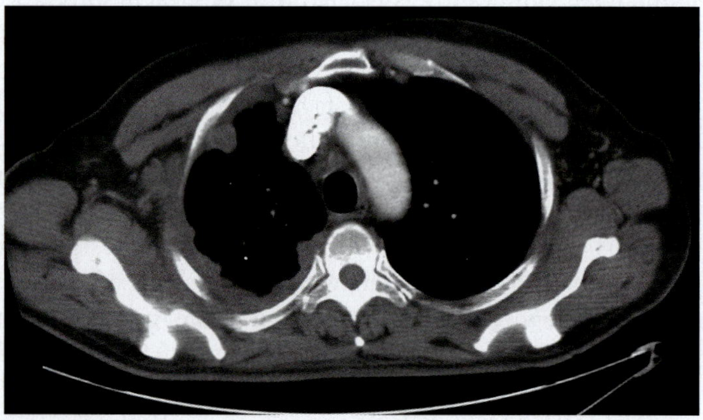

FIGURE 3-2: T2 disease. Axial CT scan showing confluent visceral pleural thickening in the right hemithorax.

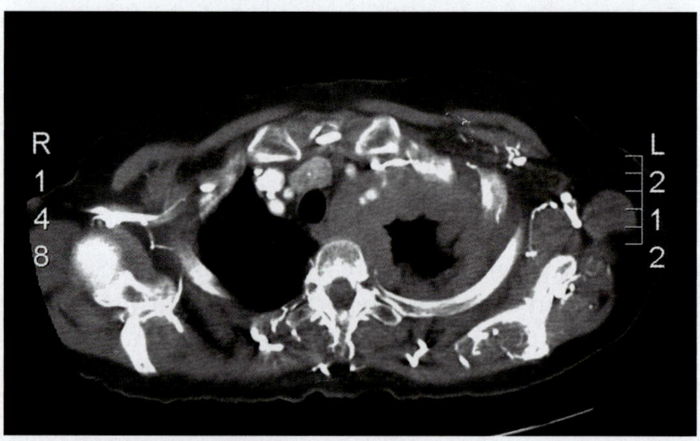

FIGURE 3-3: T4 disease. Axial CT scan showing thickened irregular pleura on the left with complete occlusion of left brachiocephalic vein and mediastinal invasion. *Note:* Contrast was injected into the left arm and entered collateral vessels in the chest wall as a result of the brachiocephalic vein occlusion.

M stage denotes the presence or absence of metastatic disease. Metastatic spread often occurs late in the course of the disease, but postmortem examinations have shown that distant spread is present in over half of pleural diffuse malignant mesothelioma patients at the time of death.[3] In some centers, aggressive debulking surgery as part of a multimodality approach is used for patients with localized resectable disease. It is vital that every effort is made to exclude metastatic disease in patients before undergoing this extensive surgical treatment.

STAGING INVESTIGATIONS IN PLEURAL DIFFUSE MALIGNANT MESOTHELIOMA

CT Scan

The introduction of multidetector row (or multislice) CT scan in the early 1990s and subsequent advances in CT scan technology significantly improved the speed and diagnostic accuracy of this imaging modality.[12] In most centers, CT scan remains the primary imaging modality used to assess disease stage, although magnetic resonance imaging (MRI) may provide additional information on T stage. A prospective study of 65 patients who underwent CT scan and MRI prior to surgical resection showed that MRI was better at identifying diaphragmatic invasion, invasion of endothoracic fascia, and solitary resectable foci of chest wall invasion.[13] The assessment of nodal status is suboptimal using CT as there is a poor correlation between nodal size and involvement with disease. Despite its limitations, the availability, speed, and relative financial economy of CT scan compared to other imaging modalities have ensured it remains an important tool for staging pleural diffuse malignant mesothelioma (Fig. 3-4).

Magnetic Resonance Imaging

Aggressive surgery is an option that is only considered in patients with early disease. Because of its inherent tissue contrast, MRI can be useful in assessing tumor invasion to identify patients with early disease.[14] Heelan et al.[13] performed a prospective trial on 65 patients who underwent contrast-enhanced CT scan and unenhanced MRI prior to a surgical procedure

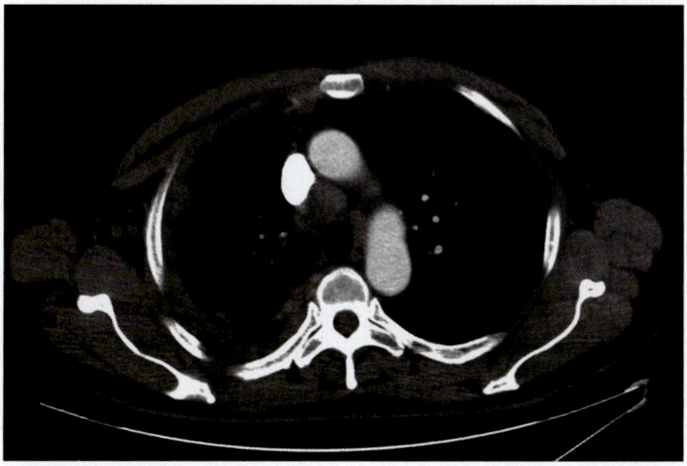

FIGURE 3-4: Axial contrast CT scan showing nodular circumferential pleural disease in the right hemithorax with malignant mediastinal nodal disease in the pre- and paratracheal areas.

(excluding percutaneous needle biopsy) to stage and/or resect the tumor. MRI was superior to CT in identifying invasion of the diaphragm (55% accuracy for CT versus 82% accuracy for MRI) and in identifying invasion of endothoracic fascia or solitary resectable foci of chest wall invasion (46% accuracy for CT versus 69% accuracy for MRI). Entwisle reported the Glenfield Hospital, UK, experience of using contrast-enhanced MRI with pleural diffuse malignant mesothelioma patients.[14] Forty-nine patients with potentially resectable disease on CT scan underwent contrast-enhanced MRI. Seventeen patients had unexpected unresectable disease demonstrated on contrast-enhanced MRI, contrast to the Heelan study finding no difference in the prediction of resectability between contrast-enhanced CT and unenhanced MRI.[13,14] Entwisle et al. propose that contrast-enhanced MRI is more accurate than unenhanced MRI when used for predicting resectability. The proportion of pleural diffuse malignant mesothelioma patients potentially suitable for aggressive surgical resection is small, and utilizing CT scan alone to estimate resectability results in up 25% of patients being upstaged at surgery.[15] If there is any doubt about the potential resectability of disease, then MRI should be considered to avoid the morbidity of unnecessary thoracotomy.

Positron Emission Tomography–Computed Tomography

The rapid evolution of technology has meant that positron emission tomography–computed tomography (PET–CT) is becoming more widely available and is being used for the investigation of malignant pleural mesothelioma (MPM) despite relatively limited data to support its use. FDG-PET has been shown to accurately delineate malignant from benign pleural disease with high sensitivity and specificity.[16] However, there remain difficulties in differentiating primary tumor extension from adjacent nodal metastases using PET–CT,[17,18] and it is not clear whether PET–CT is any better than modern CT scan or MRI in T-staging MPM. PET–CT may be most useful for detecting distant metastases in patients potentially undergoing aggressive multimodality therapy. There is some evidence that PET–CT may be better at detecting metastases than CT alone, but this is limited to small series.[19] PET–CT probably represents a significant advance in pleural diffuse malignant mesothelioma investigation but is limited by radiologically undetectable microscopic disease (false negatives) and benign inflammatory or infective conditions (false positives). PET–CT findings must be correlated with other imaging modalities, clinical history, and, if possible, histologic confirmation of FDG-avid nodes if aggressive surgery is being considered. Further studies are needed to establish the precise role of PET–CT in the staging of pleural diffuse malignant mesothelioma.

Mediastinoscopy

The usefulness of mediastinoscopy in the staging of pleural diffuse malignant mesothelioma has yet to be established. Schouwink et al.[20] performed chest CT scans and cervical mediastinoscopy in 43 patients with proven unilateral disease potentially suitable for surgical resection. CT scan and mediastinoscopy results were compared with final histopathologic findings obtained at thoracotomy. If thoracotomy was not performed, CT scan was compared to mediastinoscopy. Correlation between CT scan and mediastinoscopy was relatively poor; CT scan showed pathologic enlarged lymph nodes in 17 of 43 patients (39%), and there was histopathologic evidence of lymph node metastases at mediastinoscopy in only 11 of these patients. Lymph node metastases were diagnosed by mediastinoscopy in six patients who had no enlarged nodes on CT scan. Positive lymph nodes were found in three patients at thoracotomy after an initial negative mediastinoscopy. Rice et al.[21] reported on 85 patients with MPM who underwent preoperative staging with mediastinoscopy or endobronchial ultrasound (EBUS).[21] Thirty-eight mediastinoscopy-negative patients underwent thoracic surgery, and eighteen were found to have nodal involvement. The sensitivity and negative predictive value for mediastinoscopy were reported as 28% and 49%, respectively. While mediastinoscopy has the potential to detect mediastinal nodes in pleural diffuse malignant mesothelioma patients, its sensitivity and specificity have not been established with large prospective trials. The precise role of mediastinoscopy in disease staging therefore remains unclear.

Video-Assisted Thoracoscopic Surgery

Video-assisted thoracoscopic surgery is a useful tool for the diagnosis of pleural diffuse malignant mesothelioma, primarily determining histologic subtype for treatment stratification, but also extremely helpful in accurately identifying T1a and T1b tumors without and with visceral pleural involvement, respectively.

Endoluminal Ultrasound

The accurate staging of mediastinal nodes in patients with diffuse malignant mesothelioma is difficult. As noted above, CT scan, PET–CT, and MRI all have a relatively low sensitivity for detecting involved mediastinal nodes, and the role of mediastinoscopy has yet to be established. EBUS and esophageal endoscopic ultrasound (EUS) have been found to be accurate for nodal assessment of lung cancer and are routinely used as an aid to staging the disease.[22,23]

Rice et al.[24] reported retrospectively on the use of EBUS and EUS in the staging of pleural diffuse malignant mesothelioma. In total, 85 patients who were potential candidates for radical surgery underwent preoperative staging with mediastinoscopy and/or EBUS/EUS. Thirty-eight patients underwent EBUS, and nodal metastases were identified in 13 of 38 (34%) patients. Twenty-two EBUS-negative patients underwent surgery with nodal sampling, and there were 10 false negatives. Sensitivity and negative predictive value for EBUS were 59% and 57%, respectively.

Tournoy et al.[25] reported on a prospective study of 32 consecutive patients with proven MPM who underwent endoscopic ultrasound and fine needle aspiration (EUS-FNA) of any enlarged lymph nodes. In total, 25 patients underwent fine needle aspiration and 27 patients had mediastinoscopy. In 11 patients, a negative EUS-FNA or mediastinoscopy was not confirmed by surgical lymph node assessment because of clinical deterioration or disease progression. Twenty-one patients had positive nodal pathology: four patients with positive EUS-FNA cytology were not treated surgically. Thoracotomy with complete lymph node dissection was done in 17 (81%) patients, and 1 (6%) patient had involved mediastinal nodes. The overall prevalence of lymph node metastasis was 24%, and the sensitivity of EUS-FNA was 80% with a specificity of 100%. EBUS and EUS had higher sensitivity than either mediastinoscopy or imaging studies for detection of nodal metastases in the two studies highlighted, suggesting that EUS and/or EBUS may be useful tools in staging the mediastinum in these patients. However, both series contained limited numbers of patients, and the role of EBUS and EUS in the mediastinal staging of pleural diffuse malignant mesothelioma requires confirmation with larger trials.

Laparoscopy

Current imaging modalities cannot always determine whether a tumor is unresectable because of direct extension through the diaphragm to the peritoneal cavity. Conlon et al.[26] performed a small prospective to determine whether laparoscopy detected transdiaphragmatic tumor extension when CT findings were equivocal. Twelve of thirty-six patients considered for surgical resection with equivocal CT findings of diaphragmatic invasion underwent laparoscopy with diaphragmatic and peritoneal biopsies. Six patients had biopsy-proven transdiaphragmatic extension or peritoneal studding with tumor. The remaining six patients subsequently underwent thoracotomy, and in no case was transdiaphragmatic extension of a tumor identified. Rice et al. evaluated the role of surgical staging procedures in pleural diffuse malignant mesothelioma. One hundred and eighteen patients, deemed clinically and radiologically resectable, underwent surgical staging.[27] Laparoscopy was performed in 109 patients and peritoneal lavage in 78 patients. Ten (9.2%) patients had gross evidence of transdiaphragmatic or peritoneal involvement. Peritoneal lavage was positive for metastatic disease in 2 (2.6%) patients, neither of whom had obvious transdiaphragmatic invasion. Laparoscopy may identify transdiaphragmatic invasion in patients with pleural diffuse malignant mesothelioma, but it is not clear whether this approach is better than MRI and/or PET–CT, both of which are used in this situation.

PROBLEMS WITH PROGNOSTIC STAGING

Accurate survival stratification is precluded in existing staging systems for a number of reasons: First, stage is not an absolute survival parameter because performance status, presence/absence of symptoms, gender, age, histologic type, thrombocytosis, and other factors influence survival; second, because pathologic staging is infrequently incorporated due to the infrequency of extrapleural pneumonectomy, clinical staging remains a blunt instrument to truly appreciate the effects of histologic subtype in appropriately stratified treatment cohorts. Clinical staging is inferior to pathologic staging but remains the best assessment method available for many unresectable cases of pleural diffuse malignant mesothelioma.

SUMMARY

The staging of pleural diffuse malignant mesothelioma poses significant challenges, and there is no single modality that provides all the information necessary to direct patient management. CT scan remains the primary imaging modality used to assess disease stage but is suboptimal for assessing diaphragmatic invasion, invasion of endothoracic fascia, and nodal status. MRI is superior to CT scan in identifying invasion of the diaphragm and invasion of endothoracic fascia, but like CT scan is relatively poor at assessing nodal status. Mediastinoscopy, EBUS, and EUS may all be useful in staging the mediastinum if aggressive surgery is considered, but prospective trial data are lacking. There is some evidence that PET–CT may be better at detecting metastases than CT alone, but there are few published prospective data on the precise role of PET–CT in tumor staging. It has yet to be established whether there is a gold standard staging strategy for pleural diffuse malignant mesothelioma. Institutions typically develop staging protocols based on the local expertise available and clinical approach to patient management rather than any strong evidence base. It is important to remember that laparoscopy is unnecessary if the diagnosis is firm, and surgery is not considered a useful therapeutic option.

References

1. Richards WG. Recent advances in mesothelioma staging. *Semin Thorac Cardiovasc Surg* 2009;21:105–110.
2. Butchart EG, Ashcroft T, Barnsley WC, et al. Pleuropneumonectomy in the management of diffuse malignant mesothelioma of the pleura. Experience with 29 patients. *Thorax* 1976;31:15–24.
3. Ruffie P, Feld R, Minkin S, et al. Diffuse malignant mesothelioma of the pleura in Ontario and Quebec: a retrospective study of 332 patients. *J Clin Oncol* 1989;7:1157–1168.
4. Curran D, Sahmoud T, Therasse P, et al. Prognostic factors in patients with pleural mesothelioma: the European Organization for Research and Treatment of Cancer experience. *J Clin Oncol* 1998;16:145–152.
5. Mattson K. Natural history and clinical stage of malignant mesothelioma. *Eur J Respir Dis* 1982;63:87.
6. Dimitrov NV, McMahon S. Presentation, diagnostic methods, staging, and natural history of malignant mesothelioma. In: Antman KH, Aisner J, eds. *Asbestos-Related Disease*. Orlando, FL: Grune & Stratton; 1987:225–238.
7. Rusch VW. A proposed new international TNM staging system for malignant pleural mesothelioma. From the International Mesothelioma Interest Group. *Chest* 1995;108:1122–1128.
8. AJCC. *Cancer Staging Manual*. 6th ed. New York, NY: Springer-Verlag; 2002:180–181.
9. UICC. *TNM Classification of Malignant Tumours*. 7th ed. New York, NY: Wiley-Liss; 2009.
10. Sugarbaker DJ, Raja M. Flores MD, et al. Resection margins, extrapleural nodal status, and cell type determine post-operative long term survival in trimodality therapy of malignant pleural mesothelioma results in 183 patients. *Thorac Cardiovasc Surg* 1999;117:54–65.
11. Allen KB, Faber LP, Warren WH. Malignant pleural mesothelioma. Extrapleural pneumonectomy and pleurectomy. *Chest Surg Clin N Am* 1994;4:113–126.
12. Rydberg J, Buckwalter KA, Caldemeyer KS, et al. Multisection CT: scanning techniques and clinical applications. *Radiographics* 2000;20:1787–1806.
13. Heelan RT, Rusch VW, Begg CB, et al. Staging of malignant pleural mesothelioma: comparison of CT and MR imaging. *AJR Am J Roentgenol* 1999;172:1039–1047.
14. Entwisle J. The use of magnetic resonance imaging in malignant mesothelioma. *Lung Cancer* 2004;45(suppl 1):S69–S71.
15. Rusch VW, Rosenzweig K, Venkatraman E, et al. A phase II trial of surgical resection and adjuvant high-dose hemithoracic radiation for malignant pleural mesothelioma. *J Thorac Cardiovasc Surg* 2001;122:788–795.
16. Duysinx B, Nguyen D, Louis R, et al. Evaluation of pleural disease with 18-fluorodeoxyglucose positron emission tomography imaging. *Chest* 204;125:489–493.
17. Erasmus JJ, Truong MT, Smythe WR, et al. Integrated computed tomography- positron emission tomography in patients with potentially resectable malignant pleural mesothelioma: staging implications. *J Thorac Cardiovasc Surg* 2005;129:1364–1370.
18. Otsuka H, Terazawa K, Morita N, et al. Is FDG-PET/CT useful for managing malignant pleural mesothelioma? *J Med Invest* 2009;56:16–20.
19. Schneider DB, Clary-Macy C, Challa S, et al. Positron emission tomography with F18-fluorodeoxyglucose in the staging and preoperative evaluation of malignant pleural mesothelioma. *J Thorac Cardiovasc Surg* 2000;120:128–133.

20. Schouwink JH, Kool LS, Rutgers EJ, et al. The value of chest computer tomography and cervical mediastinoscopy in the preoperative assessment of patients with malignant pleural mesothelioma. *Ann Thorac Surg* 2003;75:1715–1718; discussion 1718–1719.
21. Rice DC, Steliga MA, Stewart J, et al. Endoscopic ultrasound-guided fine needle aspiration for staging of malignant pleural mesothelioma. *Ann Thorac Surg* 2009;88:862–868; discussion 868–869.
22. Larsen SS, Vilmann P, Krasnik M, et al. Endoscopic ultrasound guided biopsy versus mediastinoscopy for analysis of paratracheal and subcarinal lymph nodes in lung cancer staging. *Lung Cancer* 2005;48:85–92.
23. Vilmann P, Puri R. The complete "medical" mediastinoscopy (EUS-FNA + EBUS-TBNA). *Minerva Med* 2007;98:331–338.
24. Rice DC, Steliga MA, Stewart J, et al. Endoscopic ultrasound-guided fine needle aspiration for staging of malignant pleural mesothelioma. *Ann Thorac Surg* 2009;88:862–868; discussion 868–869.
25. Tournoy KG, Burgers SA, Annema JT, et al. Transesophageal endoscopic ultrasound with fine needle aspiration in the preoperative staging of malignant pleural mesothelioma. *Clin Cancer Res* 2008;14:6259–6263.
26. Conlon KC, Rusch VW, Gillern S. Laparoscopy: an important tool in the staging of malignant pleural mesothelioma. *Ann Surg Oncol* 1996;3:489–494.
27. Rice DC, Erasmus JJ, Stevens CW, et al. Extended surgical staging for potentially resectable malignant pleural mesothelioma. *Ann Thorac Surg* 2005;80:1988–92; discussion 1992–1993.

Imaging

4

▶ Jason Lester

IMAGING TECHNIQUES FOR THE DIAGNOSIS AND RADIOLOGIC STAGING OF DIFFUSE MALIGNANT MESOTHELIOMA

Various imaging techniques have an essential role in the diagnosis, staging, and assessment of treatment response in diffuse malignant mesothelioma. It is recognized that these tumors pose considerable diagnostic challenges to clinicians and radiologists. Pleural diffuse malignant mesothelioma has a unique growth pattern; it does not form discrete tumor masses but rather appears as diffuse nodular pleural thickening that can be difficult to both identify and quantify using current imaging modalities. Imaging is integral in disease management, and patients will often undergo many radiologic investigations during the course of their illness. Computed tomography (CT) scan, magnetic resonance imaging (MRI), positron emission tomography (PET), and combined PET–CT all have been used to evaluate this disease, although the relative importance of these imaging modalities has changed over time with advances in technology.[1] This chapter summarizes the current situation and highlights future advances in diagnostic imaging of pleural diffuse malignant mesothelioma.

RADIOLOGIC ASSESSMENT OF PLEURAL DIFFUSE MALIGNANT MESOTHELIOMA

A chest x-ray is the first radiologic investigation performed in the majority of patients with pleural diffuse malignant mesothelioma. Chest x-ray findings include pleural effusion (Fig. 4-1), pleural thickening, contraction of the affected hemithorax (Fig. 4-2), and, in advanced cases, chest wall invasion and rib destruction. These findings are however not specific and can be seen in a range of other benign and malignant conditions. Most patients will also undergo a CT scan of the thorax. This allows visualization of the entire pleural surface from the thoracic inlet to the level of the third lumbar vertebra. The CT appearance, taken in the context of the clinical history, will determine further investigation. Features that are helpful in distinguishing malignant from benign pleural disease are circumferential pleural thickening, nodular pleural thickening, parietal pleural thickening >1 cm, and mediastinal pleural involvement[2] (Figs. 4-3 and 4-4). However, pleural diffuse malignant mesothelioma cannot reliably be differentiated from pleural metastases on CT scan, and in the early stages of disease, differentiating benign from malignant change can be difficult. In addition, patients may previously have had pleural procedures (such as pleurodesis), which can mimic the appearance

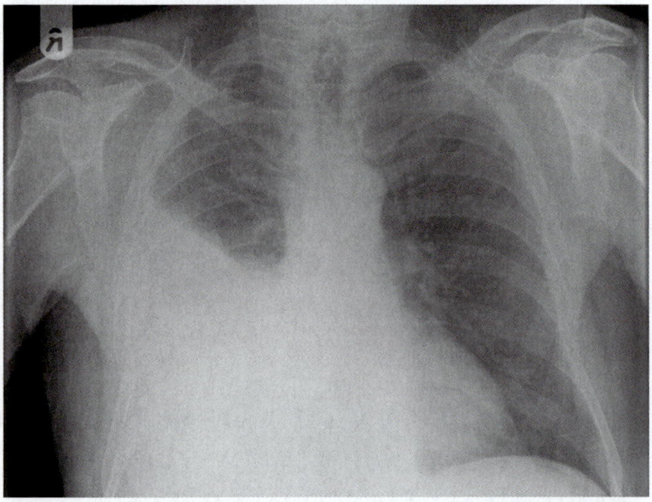

FIGURE 4-1: Chest x-ray in a patient with malignant pleural mesothelioma showing a large right-sided pleural effusion.

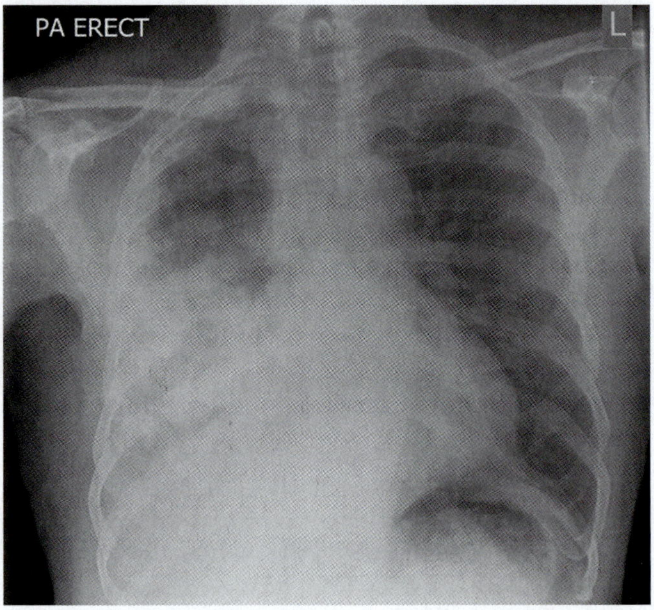

FIGURE 4-2: Chest x-ray showing contraction of the right hemithorax and pleural thickening in a patient with pleural diffuse malignant mesothelioma. Note the acute infective consolidation at the right lung base.

of pleural disease. CT scan alone is therefore not diagnostic, and histologic confirmation is required. Cytologic examination of pleural fluid classifies about 60% of malignant metastatic effusions; however, pleural diffuse malignant mesothelioma is not a diagnosis that can be rendered confidently in the vast majority of cases of pleural diffuse malignant mesothelioma. By definition, invasion cannot be assessed in exfoliative samples.[3,4] Image-guided percutaneous needle biopsy of pleural thickening is a relatively safe procedure and has been shown to be superior to Abrams pleural biopsy and has largely replaced the latter approach[5,6] (Fig. 4-5). The vast majority of cases require open biopsy for diagnosis, however.

CT scan remains the commonest modality used for evaluating treatment response in pleural diffuse malignant mesothelioma.[7,8] For solid tumors, response to treatment is usually assessed by measuring the change in longest diameter, based on the Response Evaluation Criteria in Solid Tumors (RECIST) unidimensional measurement approach.[9] For spherical tumors, there is a direct relationship between diameter and volume, and RECIST is

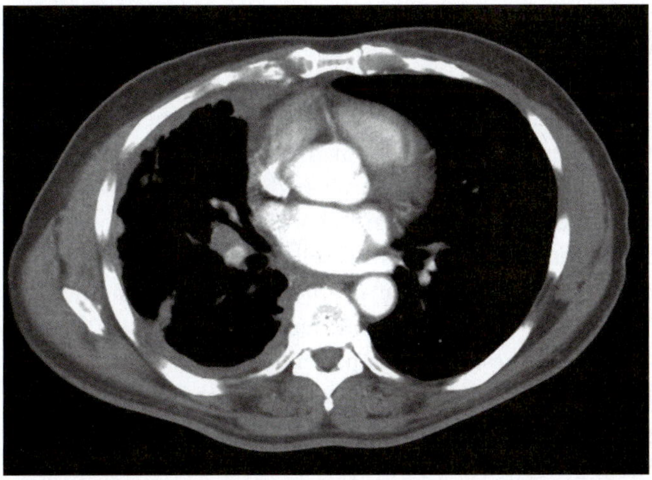

FIGURE 4-3: Contrast CT showing right-sided circumferential nodular pleural thickening in a patient with pleural diffuse malignant mesothelioma.

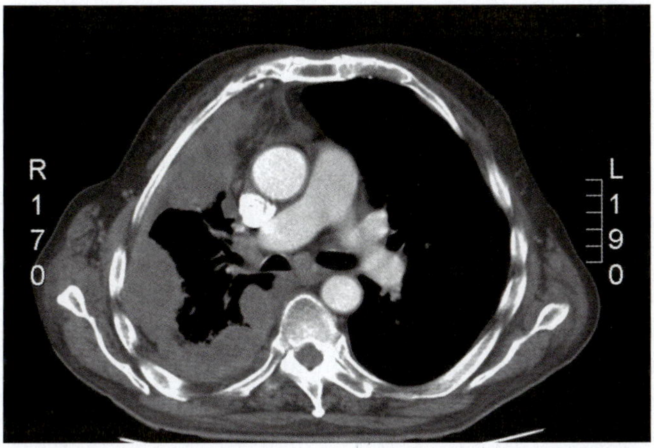

FIGURE 4-4: Contrast CT showing bulky right-sided irregular pleural thickening involving the mediastinal pleura in a patient with pleural diffuse malignant mesothelioma.

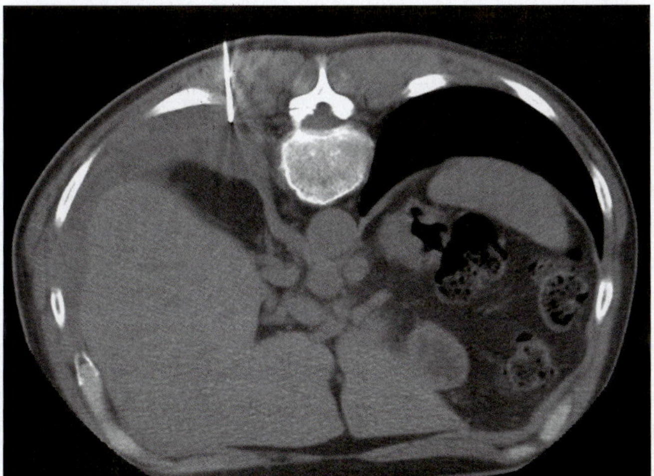

FIGURE 4-5: CT-guided biopsy of pleural thickening.

a reasonable surrogate for volume change. RECIST categorizes change in tumor diameter as progressive disease if there is an increase in diameter of at least 20%, partial response if there is a reduction in diameter of at least 30%, and stable disease for those measurement changes between these two limits. The morphology of pleural diffuse malignant mesothelioma makes the application of RECIST difficult. The tumors tend not to form discrete tumor masses like, for example, non–small cell lung cancer; instead, they appear as diffuse irregular areas of pleural thickening. As such, identifying the longest diameter to apply RECIST is problematic and often impossible (Fig. 4-3). The inadequacy of using RECIST for response evaluation is well known, and hence a modified RECIST measurement protocol where tumor thickness is measured perpendicular to the chest wall or mediastinum has been proposed.[10] Byrne et al. evaluated 73 pleural diffuse malignant mesothelioma patients from two clinical trials of cisplatin–gemcitabine chemotherapy. Tumor thickness perpendicular to the chest wall or mediastinum was measured in two positions at three separate levels on thoracic CT scans. The sum of the six measurements defined a pleural unidimensional measure. A reduction in the measurement sum of at least 30% on two occasions 4 weeks apart defined a partial response; an increase of 20% over the nadir measurement, progressive disease, and stable disease were defined as measurement changes between these two limits. Response according to these criteria predicted longer survival compared to patients with stable or progressive disease (15.1 months versus 8.9 months; $p = 0.03$). Unfortunately, modified RECIST is also unlikely to be a particularly accurate tool for assessing treatment response in patients with pleural diffuse malignant mesothelioma. First, thickness measurements perpendicular to the chest wall are subject to observer interpretation and hence intra- and interobserver variation.[11] Second, geometric modeling has shown that the application of the modified RECIST response criteria to pleural diffuse malignant mesothelioma thickness measurements yields partial response and progressive disease classifications based on much smaller volume changes than for spherical tumors.[12]

Given the stated weaknesses of linear measurements of pleural diffuse malignant mesothelioma to determine response, direct tumor volume measurement would be the most accurate approach; however, it is impractical and time-consuming without an automated system.

Computer algorithms to automatically identify and quantify pleural diffuse malignant mesothelioma tumor volumes on CT imaging are being developed to better assess therapy response.[13,14] These algorithms will need validation but may offer a more accurate and reproducible method of evaluating treatment response.

IMAGING OF PERITONEAL DIFFUSE MALIGNANT MESOTHELIOMA

The second most common site for diffuse malignant mesothelioma is the peritoneum, and although overall more men develop the disease in absolute terms, a higher proportion of women than men develop the disease in the peritoneal cavity. This is important because the female peritoneum exhibits a variety of distinct pathologic tumors unrelated to asbestos, particularly primary peritoneal mullerian-type (serous) carcinoma. CT findings include ascites and localized and diffuse omental and mesenteric masses. The diffuse pattern, characterized by thickening of the peritoneum in a sheet-like or nodular pattern, is the most common pattern and is usually of epithelioid histologic subtype. Localized masses have been suggested to more often represent sarcomatoid histologic subtype, although there is no robust correlation. Omental caking may manifest as fine, nodular tumor studding rather than multifocal nodular disease. Infiltration of the mesenteric vasculature is associated with the distinct "stellate" mesenteric pattern. Tumor infiltration of the small bowel produces abnormal fold thickening. As nodal metastases are uncommon from peritoneal diffuse malignant mesothelioma, marked lymph nodal enlargement suggests an alternate diagnosis, such as carcinomatosis, lymphomatosis, or tuberculous peritonitis.

POSITRON EMISSION TOMOGRAPHY WITH FLUORODEOXYGLUCOSE

CT remains the primary imaging modality in the staging of pleural diffuse malignant mesothelioma. It is used to assess the extent of local disease invasion, nodal involvement, and distant metastases. However, there are limitations to the utility of CT in staging pleural diffuse malignant mesothelioma. The accurate assessment of nodal status is limited due to a poor correlation between mediastinal nodal size and tumor involvement. PET, a nuclear medicine technique that produces a three-dimensional image of tissue metabolic activity, detects gamma rays emitted by a positron-emitting radionuclide (18F), which is introduced into the body on a biologically active molecule, most commonly fluorodeoxyglucose (FDG), an analogue of glucose. FDG-PET relies on the differential uptake of 18F-FDG in tissue with high metabolic activity such as most types of malignant neoplasm, compared to nonmalignant tissue.

BENIGN VERSUS MALIGNANT DISEASE

FDG-PET has been shown to accurately delineate benign from malignant pleural disease. In a prospective study of 98 consecutive patients presenting with pleural thickening or an exudative pleural effusion, an FDG-PET was performed on each patient before histologic diagnosis.[15] Sixty-three of 98 patients were found to have malignant pleural disease after histologic analysis. Sixty-one of 63 patients with histologically confirmed malignant disease showed FDG uptake within the area of pleural thickening. Only two patients with malignant pleural disease did not show increased FDG uptake. FDG-PET imaging showed an absence of FDG uptake and correctly classified 31 of 35 benign lesions. The sensitivity of FDG-PET to identify malignancy was 96.8% with a negative predictive value of 93.9%, while its specificity was 88.5% and its positive predictive value was 93.8%. Despite these impressive results, definitive diagnosis can only be achieved through histologic confirmation.

IMPLICATIONS FOR STAGING OF FDG-PET

Studies examining the role of FDG-PET in assessing nodal status are conflicting. Benard et al. evaluated 28 consecutive patients with suspected pleural diffuse malignant mesothelioma by FDG-PET imaging and found hypermetabolic lymph node involvement in 12 patients, 9 of which appeared normal on CT scan. Histologic examination in six patients confirmed malignant nodal disease in five cases.[8] However, a larger retrospective study of 63 pleural diffuse malignant mesothelioma patients (60 preoperatively and 3 to assess disease recurrence after surgery) who underwent FDG-PET reported a sensitivity of only 11% for nodal status.[16] FDG-PET undoubtedly lacks the precise anatomical imaging of CT (Figs. 4-6 to 4-8), but technologic advances have resulted in the development of PET–CT, which combines both PET and CT scanners in a single gantry system so that images acquired from both devices can be taken in the same session and combined into a single fused image.

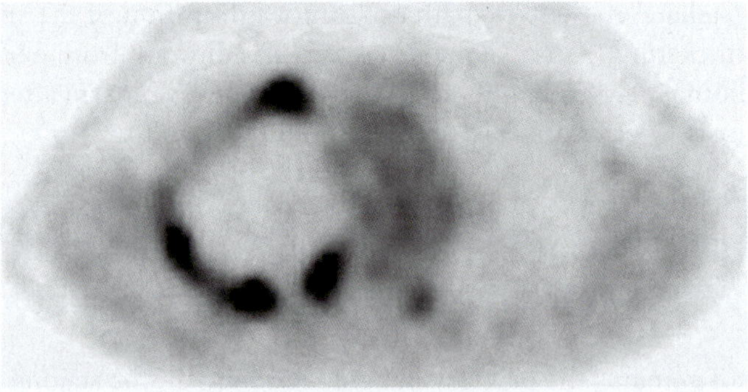

FIGURE 4-6: Axial PET image showing nodular pleural enhancement in the right hemithorax in a patient with pleural diffuse malignant mesothelioma.

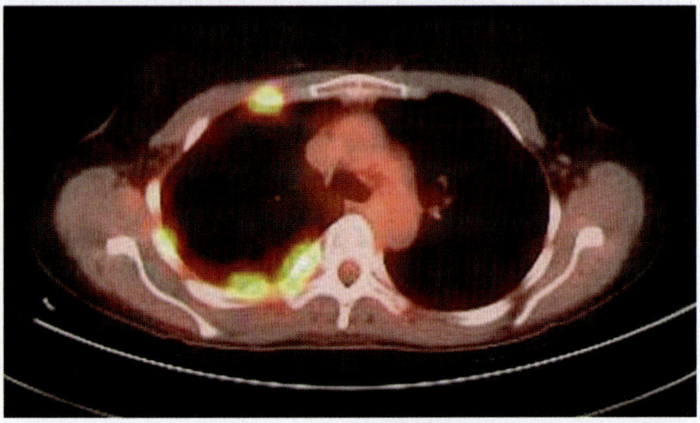

FIGURE 4-7: Axial PET–CT image. This is the image of Figure 4.6 fused with CT. Note the significantly improved anatomical definition.

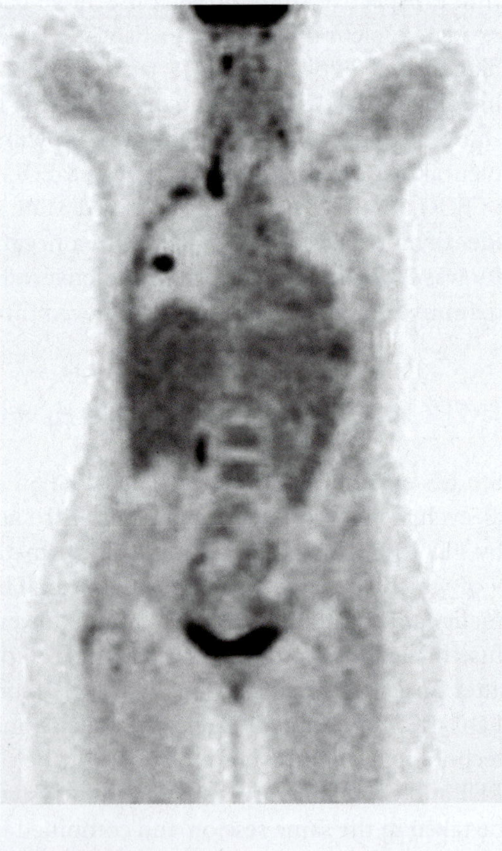

FIGURE 4-8: Coronal PET image of a patient with right pleural diffuse malignant mesothelioma showing increased uptake in the right lung pleura with nodular involvement of the horizontal fissure.

Thus, PET functional imaging can now be precisely correlated with CT anatomical imaging (Figs. 4-7 to 4-9), and as a consequence stand-alone FDG-PET scanners are no longer being manufactured. The rapid evolution of technology has made PET–CT widely available for the investigation of pleural diffuse malignant mesothelioma despite relatively limited data to support its use. There are difficulties in differentiating primary tumor extension from adjacent nodal metastases using PET–CT, but it can be useful for detecting distant metastases and for evaluating activity in supraclavicular or abdominal lymph nodes.[17,18] PET–CT probably represents a significant advance in pleural diffuse malignant mesothelioma investigation, but is limited by radiologically undetectable microscopic disease (false negatives) and benign inflammatory or infective conditions (false positives). PET–CT findings must be correlated with other imaging modalities, clinical history, and, if possible, histologic confirmation of FDG-avid nodes prior to consideration of aggressive surgery (Fig. 4-10).

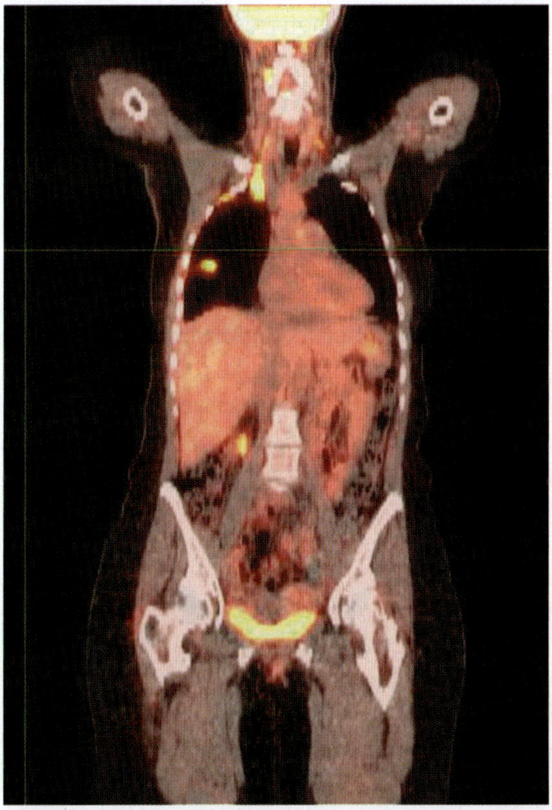

FIGURE 4-9: The same image as Figure 4-8, fused with CT scan image.

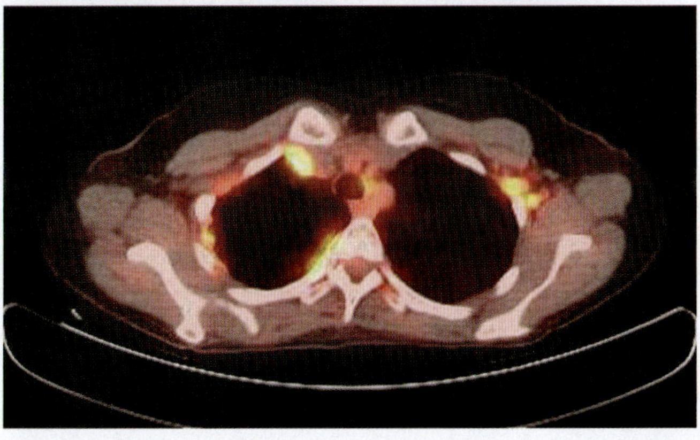

FIGURE 4-10: Axial PET–CT image of a patient with right pleural diffuse malignant mesothelioma and FDG-avid left axillary nodes, which were histologically involved with disease.

RESPONSE EVALUATION

Measuring response of pleural diffuse malignant mesothelioma to treatment is challenging because of the diffuse circumferential tumor growth pattern. FDG-PET and PET–CT are increasingly being used to assess treatment response in other tumor sites and may have a role in patients with pleural diffuse malignant mesothelioma.[19] Ceresoli et al.[20] examined 22 patients with histologically proven pleural diffuse malignant mesothelioma evaluated by FDG-PET and CT before and after two cycles of pemetrexed-based chemotherapy. A decrease of 25% or more in tumor FDG uptake as measured by standardized uptake value (SUV) was defined as a metabolic response. Of 20 patients assessable for early metabolic response with FDG-PET, 8 were classified as responders (40%) and 12 as nonresponders (60%). Early metabolic response was significantly correlated with median time to progression (14 months for metabolic responders versus 7 months for nonresponders, $p = 0.02$). No correlation was found between median time to progression and radiologic response evaluated by CT scan. A second study of 23 patients investigated quantitative volume-based FDG-PET analysis to assess treatment response.[21] Patients underwent both FDG-PET and conventional radiologic response assessment before and after one cycle of chemotherapy. Quantitative volume-based FDG-PET analysis was performed to obtain the total glycolytic volume (TGV) of the tumor. Of 23 patients suitable for both radiologic and FDG-PET analysis, 20 had CT measurable disease. After one cycle of chemotherapy, 7 patients attained a partial response and 13 had stable disease on CT by modified RECIST criteria. In the 7 patients with radiologic partial response, the median TGV on quantitative PET analysis fell to 30% of baseline (range, 11% to 71%). After one cycle of chemotherapy, a statistically significant relationship between a fall in TGV and improved patient survival was reported ($p = 0.015$). Unlike the Ceresoli study, a reduction in the SUV was not predictive of a better outcome and nor were CT measurements. Therefore, FDG-PET may have a role in predicting response to treatment and outcomes in patients with pleural diffuse malignant mesothelioma; however, larger prospective clinical trials are required to better define this role.

MAGNETIC RESONANCE IMAGING

Until recently, MRI had a clear advantage over CT in the imaging of pleural diffuse malignant mesothelioma; the multiplanar capabilities inherent to MRI allow for the acquisition of high-quality images in any plane. The growth pattern of pleural diffuse malignant mesothelioma means that coronal and sagittal imaging views are often more useful than axial views for assessing chest wall or diaphragmatic invasion. Historically, accurate CT imaging was confined to the axial plane; it was possible to reformat axial data to generate coronal and sagittal views, but these were of poor quality. The widespread introduction of multidetector row CT scanners has allowed rapid high-resolution image acquisition with no preferred plane for image reconstruction, and this increased quality of CT imaging has led to a reduction in the use of MRI for the evaluation of patients with suspected pleural diffuse malignant mesothelioma. There are however three areas where MRI can be a useful imaging modality: in the evaluation of benign versus malignant disease, for response evaluation, and for molecular imaging.

MRI can provide additional information to CT scan because of its excellent contrast resolution and can assist in the differentiation of malignant from benign pleural disease in patients with asbestos exposure.[22] Pleural diffuse malignant mesothelioma typically appears hyperintense on T2-weighted imaging and enhances following intravenous gadolinium contrast on T1-weighted images. Boraschi et al.[23] examined 30 patients with a history of asbestos exposure and pleural lesions on chest x-ray and CT who underwent MRI. A histologic diagnosis was established in all patients. Eighteen patients affected with multiple pleural plaques only showed low signal intensity on both unenhanced and enhanced T1-weighted and T2-weighted images. Eleven malignant lesions (all were diffuse malignant mesothelioma) and a solitary benign pleural plaque revealed high signal intensity on T2-weighted images and contrast enhancement in the T1-weighted images. The sensitivity and specificity of MRI in classifying a lesion as suggestive of malignancy were 100% and 95%, respectively. Typical features of pleural diffuse malignant mesothelioma on MRI are circumferential pleural thickening, pleural nodularity, irregular pleural contour, and infiltration of the chest wall or diaphragm. It is important to note that these appearances are not specific for pleural diffuse malignant mesothelioma and can be seen in other pleural malignant diseases, as well as occasionally in benign asbestos-related pleural disease. Hierholzer et al. performed retrospective study of 42 patients with pleural disease, all of whom were examined with both CT scan and MRI.[24] Using morphologic features in combination with the signal intensity features, MRI had a sensitivity of 100% and a specificity of 93% in the detection of pleural malignancy. The authors' conclusion was that when signal intensity and morphologic features are assessed, MRI is more useful and therefore superior to CT scan in differentiation of malignant from benign pleural disease. Despite the increased sensitivity and specificity of MRI in diagnosing malignant pleural disease, in practical terms where there is any suggestion of a malignant pleural process on CT scan or MRI, histologic confirmation should be obtained. For this reason, CT scan remains the radiologic investigation of choice for assessment of pleural disease.

Aggressive surgery is only considered in patients with early disease, and MRI can be useful in assessing tumor invasion because of its inherent tissue contrast.[25] Heelan et al.,[26] in a prospective trial on 65 patients who underwent contrast-enhanced CT scan and unenhanced MRI prior to a surgical procedure (excluding percutaneous needle biopsy) to stage and/or resect the tumor, found that MRI was superior to CT scan in identifying invasion of the diaphragm (55% accuracy for CT scan versus 82% accuracy for MRI) and in identifying invasion of endothoracic fascia or solitary resectable foci of chest wall invasion (46% accuracy for CT scan versus 69% accuracy for MRI). Entwisle reported the UK Leicester experience of using contrast-enhanced MRI in patients with pleural diffuse malignant mesothelioma.[25] Forty-nine patients with potentially resectable disease on CT scan underwent a contrast-enhanced MRI. Seventeen patients had unexpected unresectable disease demonstrated on contrast-enhanced MRI. This finding is in contrast to the Heelan study where no difference in the prediction of resectability was seen between contrast-enhanced CT and unenhanced MRI.[26] It is likely then that contrast-enhanced MRI is more accurate than unenhanced MRI when used for predicting resectability. What is not known is whether there is a clinical difference between contrast-enhanced CT and contrast-enhanced MRI in predicting resectability.

Dynamic contrast-enhanced-MRI (DCE-MRI) is the acquisition of sequential images during the passage of a contrast agent within a tissue of interest. Gadolinium contrast agents allow visualization of vasculature and can be used to assess vascular permeability. Recent studies have shown that the temporal evolution of gadolinium-induced signal intensity within a tumor reflects the angiogenic properties of the tumor, and these changes can be quantified and are related to vascular density and other angiogenic characteristics of lesions, such as the level of vascular endothelial growth factor, which is known to be expressed in the majority of pleural diffuse malignant mesotheliomas.[27,28] Therefore, DCE-MRI potentially provides noninvasive characterization of antiangiogenic response of pleural diffuse malignant mesothelioma to treatment.[29,30] DCE-MRI may, therefore, have a future role in assessing pleural diffuse malignant mesothelioma response to novel therapeutic agents, but further studies are needed to validate this approach.

MOLECULAR IMAGING

The introduction of new techniques, in particular PET–CT, has resulted in significant advances in pleural diffuse malignant mesothelioma imaging over recent years. Despite this, further improvements are needed for more accurate assessment of disease stage and response to treatment. Particularly, developments are needed that will allow therapy to be better tailored to the individual patients' needs and increase the accuracy of local therapies such as surgery and radiotherapy. CT scan remains the most common imaging technique used to assess treatment response and monitor disease status, but the differentiation of residual or recurrent disease from benign changes using anatomical detail alone, particularly in the postoperative setting, can be difficult.[31]

Molecular imaging is a relatively new discipline that combines molecular biology with conventional imaging modalities. Probes known as biomarkers are used to help image particular targets. Biomarkers interact chemically with their target tissue and can allow disease to be identified based on molecular rather than structural changes. Radiolabeled antibodies take advantage of the natural biochemical specificity of the immune system to provide molecularly targeted agents for cancer imaging. In principle, because antibodies can be made against virtually any biomolecule, there is opportunity to develop radiotracers that target many physiologic and pathophysiologic processes of importance to cancer biology, diagnosis, and therapy.[32] Mesothelin is a cell surface antigen that is expressed in mesothelial cells. Studies have shown that mesothelin is strongly overexpressed in almost all epithelioid diffuse malignant mesotheliomas.[33] Several other cancers, including adenocarcinoma of the lung and various nonpulmonary adenocarcinomas, also overexpress mesothelin. In contrast, there is limited expression of mesothelin in normal tissues. This makes mesothelin a potentially useful target for molecular imaging in epithelioid subtype pleural diffuse malignant mesothelioma. The monoclonal antibody K1 is a murine IgG1 that recognizes mesothelin.[34] ^{99m}Tc-labeled K1 antibodies have been developed and show promise as a potential imaging agent for pleural diffuse malignant mesothelioma. Studies are being planned to evaluate the utility of ^{99m}Tc-labeled K1 antibodies using single photon emission computed tomography as the imaging modality.

References

1. Armato SG, Entwisle J, Truong T, et al. Current state and future directions of pleural mesothelioma imaging. *Lung Cancer* 2008;59:411–420.
2. Leung AN, Muller NL, Miller RR. CT in differential diagnosis of diffuse pleural disease. *AJR Am J Roentgenol* 1990;154:487–492.
3. Pedio G, Landolt-Weber U. Cytologic presentation of malignant mesothelioma in pleural effusions. *Exp Cell Biol* 1988;56:211–216.
4. Renshaw AA, Dean BR, Antman KH, et al. The role of cytologic evaluation of pleural fluid in the diagnosis of malignant mesothelioma. *Chest* 1997;111:106–109.

5. Adams RF, Gray W, Davies RJ, et al. Percutaneous image-guided cutting needle biopsy of the pleura in the diagnosis of malignant mesothelioma. *Chest* 2001;120:1798–1802.
6. Maskell NA, Gleeson FV, Davies RJ. Standard pleural biopsy versus CT-guided cutting-needle biopsy for diagnosis of malignant disease in pleural effusions: a randomised controlled trial. *Lancet* 2003;361:1326–1330.
7. Rydberg J, Buckwalter KA, Caldemeyer KS, et al. Multisection CT: scanning techniques and clinical applications. *Radiographics* 2000;20:1787–1806.
8. Bénard F, Sterman D, Smith RJ, et al. Metabolic imaging of malignant pleural mesothelioma with fluorodeoxyglucose positron emission tomography. *Chest* 1998;114:713–722.
9. Therasse P, Arbuck SG, Eisenhauer EA, et al. New guidelines to evaluate the response to treatment in solid tumors. European Organization for Research and Treatment of Cancer, National Cancer Institute of the United States, National Cancer Institute of Canada. *J Natl Cancer Inst* 2000;92:205–216.
10. Byrne MJ, Nowak AK. Modified RECIST criteria for assessment of response in malignant pleural mesothelioma. *Ann Oncol* 2004;15:257–260.
11. Armato SG III, Oxnard GR, MacMahon H, et al. Measurement of mesothelioma on thoracic CT scans: a comparison of manual and computer-assisted techniques. *Med Phys* 2004;31:1105–1115.
12. Oxnard GR, Armato SG III, Kindler HL. Modeling of mesothelioma growth demonstrates weaknesses of current response criteria. *Lung Cancer* 2006;52:141–148.
13. Armato SG III, Oxnard GR, Kocherginsky M, et al. Evaluation of semiautomated measurements of mesothelioma tumor thickness on CT scans. *Acad Radiol* 2005;12:1301–1309.
14. Zhao B, Schwartz LH, Flores R, et al. Automated segmentation of mesothelioma volume on CT scan. *SPIE Proc* 2005;5747:866–871.
15. Duysinx B, Nguyen D, Louis R, et al. Evaluation of pleural disease with 18-fluorodeoxyglucose positron emission tomography imaging. *Chest* 2004;125:489–493.
16. Flores RM, Akhurst T, Gonen M, et al. Positron emission tomography defines metastatic disease but not locoregional disease in patients with malignant pleural mesothelioma. *J Thorac Cardiovasc Surg* 2003;126:11–16.
17. Erasmus JJ, Truong MT, Smythe WR, et al. Integrated computed tomography-positron emission tomography in patients with potentially resectable malignant pleural mesothelioma: staging implications. *J Thorac Cardiovasc Surg* 2005;129:1364–1370.
18. Otsuka H, Terazawa K, Morita N, et al. Is FDG-PET/CT useful for managing malignant pleural mesothelioma? *J Med Invest* 2009;56:16–20.
19. Eary JF. PET imaging for treatment response in cancer. *PET Clin* 2008;3:101–109.
20. Ceresoli GL, Chiti A, Zucali PA, et al. Early response evaluation in malignant pleural mesothelioma by positron emission tomography with [18F]fluorodeoxyglucose. *J Clin Oncol* 2006;24:4587–4593.
21. Francis RJ, Byrne MJ, van der Schaaf AA, et al. Early prediction of response to chemotherapy and survival in malignant pleural mesothelioma using a novel semiautomated 3-dimensional volume-based analysis of serial 18F-FDG PET scans. *J Nucl Med* 2007;48:1449–1458.
22. Knuuttila A, Halme M, Kivisaari L, et al. The clinical importance of magnetic resonance imaging versus computed tomography in malignant pleural mesothelioma. *Lung Cancer* 1998;22:215–225.
23. Boraschi P, Neri S, Braccini G, et al. Magnetic resonance appearance of asbestos-related benign and malignant pleural diseases. *Scand J Work Environ Health* 1999;25:18–23.
24. Hierholzer J, Luo L, Bittner RC, et al. MRI and CT in the differential diagnosis of pleural disease. *Chest* 2000;118:604–609.
25. Entwisle J. The use of magnetic resonance imaging in malignant mesothelioma. *Lung Cancer* 2004;45(suppl 1):S69–S71.
26. Heelan RT, Rusch VW, Begg CB, et al. Staging of malignant pleural mesothelioma: comparison of CT and MR imaging. *AJR Am J Roentgenol* 1999;172:1039–1047.
27. Strizzi L, Catalano A, Vianale G, et al. Vascular endothelial growth factor is an autocrine growth factor in human malignant mesothelioma. *J Pathol* 2001;193:468–475.
28. Aoe K, Hiraki A, Tanaka T, et al. Expression of vascular endothelial growth factor in malignant mesothelioma. *Anticancer Res* 2006;26:4833–4836.

29. Knopp MV, Giesel FL, Marcos H, et al. Dynamic contrast-enhanced magnetic resonance imaging in oncology. *Top Magn Reson Imaging* 2001;12:301–308.
30. Yamamuro M, Gerbaudo VH, Gill RR, et al. Morphologic and functional imaging of malignant pleural mesothelioma. *Eur J Radiol* 2007;64:356–366.
31. Steinert HC, Santos Dellea MM, Burger C, et al. Therapy response evaluation in malignant pleural mesothelioma with integrated PET-CT imaging. *Lung Cancer* 2005;49(suppl 1):S33–S35.
32. Kelloff GJ, Krohn KA, Larson SM, et al. The progress and promise of molecular imaging probes in oncologic drug development. *Clin Cancer Res* 2005;11:7967–7985.
33. Ordonez NG. Value of mesothelin immunostaining in the diagnosis of mesothelioma. *Mod Pathol* 2003;16:192–197.
34. Hassan R, Wu C, Brechbiel MW, et al. 111Indium-labeled monoclonal antibody K1: biodistribution study in nude mice bearing a human carcinoma xenograft expressing mesothelin. *Intl J Cancer* 1999;80:559–563.

Non–Asbestos-Related Diffuse Malignant Mesothelioma

5

Allen R. Gibbs
Richard L. Attanoos

There is overwhelming epidemiologic and mineralogic evidence showing amphiboles as the cause of the vast majority of diffuse malignant mesothelioma in men. Approximately 80% of diffuse malignant mesotheliomas are thought to be caused by exposure to asbestos. The relationship between asbestos and diffuse malignant mesothelioma is well known and has been extensively examined.

There are, however, compelling reasons to also accept that diffuse malignant mesothelioma and asbestos are not invariably associated. There is good evidence to support the existence of non–asbestos-related diffuse malignant mesothelioma. These factors are reviewed below. Sporadic or spontaneous diffuse malignant mesothelioma is discussed in Chapter 6.

Genetic factors predisposing to diffuse malignant mesothelioma are suspected to underpin the existence of familial clusterings in communities—some exist in asbestos-exposed households and some appear unrelated to asbestos. Genetic polymorphisms of carcinogen deactivating genes (such as glutathione *S*-transferase) may play a role in individual susceptibility to diffuse malignant mesothelioma.

FIBROUS ZEOLITE (ERIONITE)

After a government nationwide survey to locate and treat residual pockets of tuberculosis in Turkey in the early 1970s, it was noted that there was a high incidence of diffuse malignant mesothelioma in certain Turkish villages in Cappadocia.[1–3] The nonoccupational nature of the exposure was suggested by the tumors occurring at a relatively young age and in women as well as men. The proportional mortality from mesothelioma was found to be 42.9% of deaths, considerably higher than previously described for any asbestos cohort.

The occurrence of mesothelioma in this region has been linked to environmental exposures to volcanic tuff containing inhalable sized fibers of erionite, a fibrous zeolite.[4,5] The inhabitants of these villages had frequently carved their homes and other structures out of soft tuff outcroppings or have cut pieces from the tuffs and transported them to sites for erection of buildings. Sometimes the tuffs were ground and used as stucco pastes and whitewashes.[6,7]

Erionite fibers have similarities to amphibole asbestos fibers, are biopersistent, and have a high internal surface area.[8] A number of animal studies were conducted to determine if erionite fiber was the agent involved in the induction of diffuse malignant mesotheliomas observed in the Cappadocian villages.[9] The high surface area appears to increase the mesothelioma potency with respect to amphibole asbestos fibers both experimentally and epidemiologically.[10] Erionite fibers have been identified in bronchoalveolar lavage samples and lung tissues of individuals with and without diffuse malignant mesothelioma living in these villages.[11,12] Familial clusterings have been reported and suggest genetic susceptibility in certain individuals.

FLUORO-EDENITE

A cluster of diffuse malignant mesothelioma was observed in Biancavilla, Sicily, Italy, in a mortality survey of diffuse malignant mesothelioma in Italy from 1988 to 1992.[13] Biancavilla is located in a volcanic area in eastern Sicily where industrial use of asbestos was not conducted. An environmental study suggested the possible cause to be usage of materials from stone quarries located near the town that contained nonasbestos fibrous amphiboles.[14] These materials were widely used in the local building industry. Mineralogic studies demonstrated that the amphibole was a fluoro-edenite, which has similar morphology and size to certain amphibole forms of asbestos.[15] It was identified in a high proportion of the samples taken from buildings in the area.[14–16] It was also identified in the lung tissues from a diffuse malignant mesothelioma case.[14] Lung specimens from 8 out of 27 sheep who lived in the area were found to have fluoro-edenite fibers.[17] Therefore, there is a consistency of evidence that exposure to fluoro-edenite mineral fibers can result in the development of diffuse malignant mesothelioma.

RADIATION

Ionizing radiation has been recognized as a human carcinogen and an established risk factor for several different types of cancer. These have included hematologic malignancies and solid tumors. In addition, there have been increasing reports of cases of pleural, pericardial, and peritoneal diffuse malignant mesothelioma that have been linked to therapeutic irradiation and thorium dioxide administration. Most postirradiation diffuse malignant mesotheliomas have followed treatment for a previous neoplasm, most frequently Hodgkin lymphoma, non-Hodgkin lymphoma, Wilms tumor, breast carcinoma, and testicular cancers.[18–23] In the Tward et al.[21] study, which followed non-Hodgkin lymphoma patients from 1973 to 2001, there was a significantly increased rate of diffuse malignant mesothelioma in patients treated with radiation compared with those which did not receive radiation.

The evidence linking ionizing radiation with the development of diffuse malignant mesothelioma has come from three types of exposure: (1) exposure to the diagnostic contrast medium "Thorotrast," which contains thorium dioxide; (2) case reports and large-scale retrospective cohort studies that have examined patients undergoing radiation treatment for previous malignant tumors; and (3) workers in the atomic energy/nuclear engineering industry.[24]

Sanders and Jackson studied the effects of intraperitoneal injection of $^{239}PuO_2$ particles into rats and found that 27% of the rats developed epithelioid diffuse malignant mesothelioma and 38% sarcomatoid diffuse malignant mesothelioma.[25]

The occurrence of diffuse malignant mesothelioma following radiation treatment for various cancers does not appear to be explained by asbestos exposure as there appeared to be no difference in asbestos exposure between patients treated by radiotherapy and those not receiving radiation treatment; for the younger patients treated with radiotherapy, there was little opportunity for asbestos exposure, and the male to female ratio is 1:1.[19,24,26]

Elevated rates of diffuse malignant mesothelioma have been reported in workers who have been occupationally exposed to radiation including external γ-ray and internal deposition of radionuclides that deliver dose primarily to the lung and lymphatic system.[27–29] Risk of developing diffuse malignant mesothelioma was elevated in employees who worked for the British Atomic Energy Authority between 1946 and 1996.[30] It was elevated in workers at the Idaho National Engineering and Environmental Laboratory where nuclear material chemical processing, construction, and demolition occurred.[31] In the largest cohort study of radiation workers in the nuclear industries in 15 countries, Cardis et al.[28] reported 39 cases of pleural cancer although this did not reach statistical significance. However, the excess relative risk for pleural cancer was one of the highest among all the cancers examined in the study. In several of the studies, there appeared to be a dose–response relationship between radiation exposure and the risk of diffuse malignant mesothelioma.

Thorotrast, a radiographic contrast medium used primarily between 1930 and 1955, contained thorium dioxide and has been linked to the development of diffuse malignant mesothelioma. Thorium dioxide is insoluble and once injected cannot be excreted but is retained within various organs including lung and pleura. It decays very slowly with the emission predominantly of α particles. Maurer and Egloff[32] described peritoneal diffuse malignant mesothelioma occurring in a non–asbestos-exposed patient 36 years after contamination of the peritoneal cavity with thorium dioxide from a cholangiogram. Dahlgren[33] described diffuse malignant mesothelioma occurring in the cervical pleura 25 years after the patient had been injected with Thorotrast for cerebral angiography. The development of peritoneal diffuse malignant mesothelioma in a 63-year-old male who had no history of asbestos exposure was linked to Thorotrast exposure that took place in 1945.[34] Cohort studies of patients who were administered Thorotrast in Denmark, Sweden, Japan, Germany, and the United States have been found to have an increased risk of diffuse malignant mesothelioma predominantly within the pleura and peritoneum.[23,35–38] In studies by Andersson et al.[35,36] and Travis et al.,[38,39] it was found that the risk increased with increasing cumulative radiation dose. The largest cohort of Thorotrast-exposed subjects was Portuguese and comprised over 2000 patients. Diffuse malignant mesothelioma was not noted as a cause of death in this cohort, but there was considerable uncertainty with respect to the cause of death in this study.[40] Therefore, overall there is a consistency in these studies, which shows that there is a risk of developing pleural and peritoneal diffuse malignant mesothelioma following Thorotrast exposure.[41]

Initially there were a number of case reports, which suggested an association between the administration of therapeutic irradiation and the development of diffuse malignant mesothelioma in serosal tissues in proximity to the fields of irradiation.[24,26] Later several large-scale retrospective cohort studies were published, which examined the development of diffuse malignant mesothelioma following therapeutic irradiation for a number of different cancers including Hodgkin lymphoma, non-Hodgkin lymphoma, breast carcinoma, and testicular carcinoma.[19–23,27–29,42–44]

Until 1996, the reported median latency between the radiation exposure to the development of the diffuse malignant mesothelioma was approximately 19.5 years with a range of 5 to 41 years.[18] This is somewhat shorter than for asbestos-induced diffuse malignant mesothelioma. In the De Bruin et al.[22] study, the median time from radiotherapy for Hodgkin lymphoma to diffuse malignant mesothelioma diagnosis was 27.7 years, with a range of 10.5 to 34.1 years. The risk of diffuse malignant mesothelioma was much more pronounced among women compared with men, among patients treated at a younger age, and after prolonged follow-up. Teta et al.[19] examined lymphoma patients and found that the average time from treatment with radiation to the diagnosis of diffuse malignant mesothelioma was 16 years for Hodgkin lymphoma and 7 years for non-Hodgkin lymphoma.

The shorter latency period for diffuse malignant mesothelioma after radiation could be explained by direct damage to the mesothelial cells and reduced immune surveillance in association with the primary tumors.

MAN-MADE VITREOUS FIBERS

With the exception of refractory ceramic fibers, most man-made vitreous fibers have low biopersistence and no confirmed potency for the development of diffuse malignant mesothelioma. Animal inhalational experiments have demonstrated potency for refractory ceramic fibers to induce diffuse malignant mesothelioma in rodents.[45] There is tentative link between refractory ceramic fibers and pleural plaques, although a conclusive link is yet to be confirmed because of the common association of confounding fibers (amphiboles) in analyzed lungs.[46]

ORGANIC FIBERS

There are anecdotal links of mesothelioma to exposure to organic fibers in the sugarcane industry, but these are not substantiated.[47]

CARBON NANOTUBES

The role of multiwalled carbon nanotubes in simulating asbestos-induced tissue injury has been recently investigated.[48,49] Both carbon nanotubes and asbestos possess similar morphologic characteristics. Long straight nanotubes and amphibole fibers were identified to induce mesothelial cell injury via cell damage and chronic inflammatory effects adjacent to mesothelial stomata, potentially a key first step in the understanding of how biopersistent respirable amphibole asbestos reach the parietal pleura in humans and induce diffuse malignant mesothelioma. There is insufficient basis to conclude that carbon nanotubes induce diffuse malignant mesothelioma in human beings.

MISCELLANEOUS

Diffuse malignant mesothelioma has been reported in association with certain chronic inflammatory processes such as empyema, posttherapeutic pneumothorax, and chronic peritonitis.[50,51] Preexisting tuberculous pleuritis has been reported decades prior to the development of diffuse malignant mesothelioma.

References

1. Artvinli M, Baris YI. Malignant mesothelioma in a small village in the Anatolian region of Turkey: an epidemiologic study. *J Natl Cancer Inst* 1979;63:17–22.
2. Baris YI, Sahin AA, Ozesmi M, et al. An outbreak of pleural mesothelioma and chronic fibrosing pleurisy in the village of Karain/Urgup in Anatolia. *Thorax* 1978;33:181–192.

3. Baris YI. Fibrous zeolite (erionite) related diseases in Turkey. *Am J Ind Med* 1991;19:373–378.
4. Dogan AU. Malignant mesothelioma and erionite. In: Pass HI, Vogelzang NJ, Carbone M, eds. *Malignant Mesothelioma.* New York, NY: Springer; 2005:242–258.
5. Pooley FD. Evaluation of fiber samples taken from the vicinity of two villages in Turkey. In: Dement R, Dement JH, eds. *Dust and Disease.* Park Forest South, IL: Pathotox Publication; 1979:41.
6. Ross M, Nolan RP, Langer AM, et al. Health effects of mineral dusts other than asbestos. In: Guthrie GD, Mossman BT, eds. *Health Effects of Mineral Dusts.* Washington, DC: Mineralogical Society of North America; 1993;361–407.
7. Rohl AN, Langer AM, Moncure G, et al. Endemic pleural disease associated with exposure to mixed fibrous dust in Turkey. *Science* 1982;216:518–520.
8. Dogan AU, Dogan M, Hoskins JA. Erionite series minerals: mineralogical and carcinogenic properties. *Environ Geochem Health* 2008;30:367–381.
9. Wagner JC, Skidmore JW, Hill RJ, et al. Erionite exposure and mesothelioma in rats. *Br J Cancer* 1985;51:727–730.
10. Coffin DL, Peters SE, Palekar LD, et al. A study of the biological activity of erionite in relation to its chemical and structural characteristics. In: Wehner AP, ed. *Biological Interaction of Inhaled Mineral Fibres and Cigarette Smoke.* Columbus, OH: Battelle Memorial Institution; 1989:313–323.
11. Sebastein P, Gauduchet A, Bignon J, et al. Ferruginous bodies in sputum as an indication of exposure to airborne mineral fibres in the mesothelioma villages of Cappadocia. *Arch Environ Health* 1981;39:18–23.
12. Dumortier P, Coplu L, Emri S, et al. Erionite bodies and fibres in bronchoalveolar lavage fluid (BALF) of residents from Tuzkoy, Cappadocia, Turkey. *Occup Environ Med* 2001;58: 261–266.
13. Di Paola M, Mastrantonio M Carboni M, et al. La mortalita per tumour malign della pleura in Italia negli anni 1988–1992. Rapporti ISTIS-AN 1996.
14. Paoletti L, Batisti D, Bruno C, et al. Unusually high incidence of malignant pleural mesothelioma in a town of eastern Sicily: an epidemiological and environmental study. *Arch Environ Heath* 2000;55:392–398.
15. Comba P, Gianfagna A, Paoletti L. Pleural mesothelioma cases in Biancavilla are related to a new fluoro-edenite fibrous amphibole. *Arch Environ Health* 2003;58:229–232.
16. Gianfagna A, Oberti R. Fluoro-edenite from Biancavilla (Catania, Sicily, Italy). Crystal chemistry of a new amphibole end-member. *Am Mineral* 2001;86:1493–1498.
17. DeNardo P, Bruni B, Paoletti L, et al. Pulmonary fibre burden in sheep living in the Biancavilla area (Sicily): preliminary results. *Sci Total Environ* 2004;325:51–58.
18. Cavazza A, Travis LB, Travis WD, et al. Post-irradiation malignant mesothelioma. *Cancer* 1996;77:1379–1385.
19. Teta MJ, Lau E, Sceurman BK, et al. Therapeutic radiation for lymphoma: risk of mesothelioma. *Cancer* 2007;109:1432–1438.
20. Hodgson DC, Gilbert ES, Dores GM, et al. Long-term solid cancer risk among 5-year survivors of Hodgkin's lymphoma. *J Clin Oncol* 2007;25:1489–1497.
21. Tward JD, Wendland MM, Shrieve DC, et al. The risk of secondary malignancies over 30 years after the treatment of non-Hodgkin lymphoma. *Cancer* 2006;107:108–115.
22. De Bruin ML, Burgers JA, Baas P, et al. Malignant mesothelioma after radiation treatment for Hodgkin lymphoma. *Blood* 2009;113:3679–3681.
23. Travis LB, Fossa SD, Schonfeld SJ, et al. Second cancer among 40576 testicular cancer patients: focus on long term survivors. *J Natl Cancer Inst* 2005;97:1354–1365.
24. Goodman JE, Nascarella MA, Valberg PA. Ionizing radiation: a risk factor for mesothelioma. *Cancer Causes Control* 2009;20:1237–1254.
25. Sanders CL, Jackson TA. Induction of mesotheliomas and sarcomas from "hot spots" of $^{239}PuO_2$ activity. *Health Phys* 1972;22:755–759.
26. Witherby SM, Butnor KJ, Grunberg SM. Malignant mesothelioma following thoracic radiotherapy for lung cancer. *Lung Cancer* 2007;57:410–413.

27. National Research Council, Committee on the Biological Effects of Ionizing Health Radiations (NRC). Risks from exposure to low levels of ionizing radiation: BEIR VII-Phase 2. Washington DC: National Academy Press; 2006.
28. Cardis E, Richardson D. Health effects of radiation exposure at uranium processing facilities. *J Radiol Prot* 2000;20:95–97.
29. Cardis E, Vrijheid M, Blettner M et al. The 15-country collaborative study of cancer risk among radiation workers in the nuclear industry: estimates of radiation-related cancer risks. *Radiat Res* 2007;167:396–416.
30. Atkinson WD, Law DV, Bromley KJ, et al. Mortality of employees of the United Kingdom Atomic Energy Authority, 1946–1997. *Occup Environ Med* 2004;61:577–585.
31. National Institute for Occupational Safety and Health (NIOSH). An epidemiologic study of mortality and radiation-related risk of cancer among workers at the Idaho National Engineering and Environmental Laboratory. HHS (NIOSH) Publ no 2005-131. 2005.
32. Maurer R, Egloff B. Malignant peritoneal mesothelioma after cholangiography with thorotrast. *Cancer* 1975;36:1381–1385.
33. Dahlgren S. Effects of locally deposited colloidal thorium dioxide. *Ann NY Acad Sci* 1967;145: 786–790.
34. Stey C, Landolt-Weber U, Vetter W, et al. Malignant peritoneal mesothelioma after Thorotrast exposure. *Am J Clin Oncol* 1995;18:313–317.
35. Andersson M, Carstensen B, Storm HH. Mortality and cancer incidence after cerebral angiography with or without Thorotrast. *Radiat Res* 1995;142:305–320.
36. Andersson M, Wallin H, Johnson M, et al. Lung carcinoma and malignant mesothelioma in patients exposed to Thorotrast. *Int J Cancer* 1995;63:330–336.
37. Ishikawa Y, Mori T, Machinami R. Lack of apparent excess in malignant mesothelioma but increased overall malignancies of peritoneal cavity in Japanese autopsies with Thorotrast injection into blood vessels. *J Cancer Res Clin Oncol* 1995;121:567–570.
38. Travis LB, Land CE, Andersson M, et al. Mortality after cerebral angiography with or without radioactive Thorotrast: an international cohort of 3, 143 two-year survivors. *Radiat Res* 2001;156: 136–150.
39. Travis LB, Hauptmann M, Gaul LK, et al. Site specific cancer incidence and mortality after cerebral angiography with radioactive Thorotrast. *Radiat Res* 2003;160:691–706.
40. Dos Santos Silva I, Malveiro F, Jones ME, et al. Mortality after radiological investigation with radioactive Thorotrast: a follow-up study of up to fifty years in Portugal. *Radiat Res* 2003;159:521–534.
41. Van Kaick G, Dalheimer A, Hornik S, et al. The German Thorotrast study: recent results and assessment of risks. *Radiat Res* 1999;152 (suppl 6):S64–S71.
42. Neugut AI, Ahsan H, Antman KH. Incidence of malignant mesothelioma after thoracic radiotherapy. *Cancer* 1997;80:948–950.
43. Brown LM, Chen BE, Pfeiffer RM, et al. Risk of second non-haematological malignancies among 376,825 breast cancer survivors. *Breast Cancer Res Treat* 2007;106:439–451.
44. Deutsch M, Land SR, Begovic M, Cecchini R, et al. An association between postoperative radiotherapy for primary breast cancer in 11 National Surgical Adjuvant Breast and Bowel Project (NSABP) studies and the subsequent appearance of malignant mesothelioma. *Am J Clin Oncol* 2007;30:294–296.
45. McConnell EE, Mast RW, Hesterberg TW, et al. Chronic inhalation toxicity of a kaolin based refractory ceramic fiber in Syrian golden hamsters. *Inhalation Toxicol* 1995;7:503–532.
46. Lockey J, Lemasters G, Rice C. Refractory ceramic fibers and pleural plaques. *Am J Respir Crit Care Med* 1996;154:1405–1410.
47. Newman RH. Fine biogenic particulate silica fibres in sugarcane: a possible hazard. *Ann Occup Hyg* 1986;30:365–370.
48. Donaldson K, Murphy FA, Duffin R, et al. Asbestos, carbon nanotubes and the pleural mesothelium: a review of the hypothesis regarding the role of long fiber retention in the parietal pleura. *Part Fibre Toxicol* 2010;7:5.

49. Murphy FA, Poland CA, Duffin R, et al. Length-dependent retention of carbon nanotubes in the pleural space of mice initiates sustained inflammation and progressive fibrosis on the parietal pleura. *Am J Pathol* 2011;178:2587–2600.
50. Hillerdal G, Berg J. Malignant mesothelioma secondary to chronic inflammation and old scars: 2 scars and a review of the literature. *Cancer* 1985;55:1968–1972.
51. Riddell RH, Goodman MJ, Moosa AR. Peritoneal malignant mesothelioma in a patient with recurrent peritonitis. *Cancer* 1981;48:134–139.

6 Spontaneous/Idiopathic Diffuse Malignant Mesothelioma

Allen R. Gibbs

The mining and milling of asbestos began in the 1890s, peaked in the early 1970s, and declined rapidly thereafter because of the recognition of the cancer hazard. The association of asbestos exposure and diffuse malignant mesothelioma was first established by Wagner and coinvestigators in 1960.[1] However, despite some assertions to the contrary by Mark and Yokoi,[2] not all diffuse malignant mesotheliomas are caused by asbestos exposure. If all diffuse malignant mesotheliomas were caused by asbestos, then the same would be a *unique* tumor in which a single cause is invariably ascribed. In fact, there is good evidence that there is a background rate of diffuse malignant mesothelioma that is not related to asbestos exposure. The evidence includes the following: (1) in some countries the rate for diffuse malignant mesothelioma in women, who would have been far less exposed to asbestos than men, has remained constant over time; (2) cases of diffuse malignant mesothelioma occur in which despite extensive investigation no history of asbestos exposure can be identified and mineral fiber analysis of lung tissues reveals background rates of mineral fibers; (3) the spontaneous occurrence of diffuse malignant mesothelioma in children and adolescents below the latent period for asbestos-related diffuse malignant mesothelioma; (4) descriptions of diffuse malignant mesothelioma occurring in individuals prior to the industrial use of asbestos; and (5) the spontaneous occurrence of diffuse malignant mesothelioma in certain animals, both wild and domesticated.[3–7]

A number of studies have reported a wide range of percentages for the association of diffuse malignant mesothelioma with asbestos exposure. Ratzer et al.[8] studied 31 cases of diffuse malignant mesothelioma and found asbestos exposure in only 13%. Borow et al.[9] reviewed 72 cases of diffuse malignant mesothelioma and found that all 60 patients for whom an exposure history was available were exposed to asbestos. Ninety-nine percent of the 70 cases studied by Cochrane and Webster[10] had an asbestos exposure history. Tagnon and coinvestigators studied 61 cases of diffuse malignant mesothelioma and found that 80% of the 55 patients with an exposure history were exposed to asbestos.[11] Oels et al.,[12] Brenner et al.,[13] and Newhouse and Thompson[14] reported asbestos exposure in 27%, 13%, and 44% of cases, respectively. Peto et al.[15] collected a series of 116 men with diffuse malignant mesothelioma in Los Angeles County and, through interviews with the patients or close relatives, found that 68% reported exposures to asbestos, 22% reported no exposure to asbestos, and in 10% asbestos exposure could not be determined. A study of 668 diffuse malignant mesotheliomas in Canada and the United States from 1960 to 1975 revealed that asbestos exposure was present in 50% of the men and only 5% of women.[16] Spirtas et al.[17] performed a case–control study of 208 US diffuse malignant mesothelioma cases and used telephone interviews with next of kin to ascertain patterns of asbestos exposure. Among men with pleural diffuse malignant mesothelioma, they found the attributable risk to asbestos exposure to be

88%, but only 58% for peritoneal mesothelioma. For women (pleural and peritoneal), the attributable risk for exposure to asbestos was 23%. In France, through the French National Mesothelioma Surveillance Program, the calculated risk of diffuse malignant mesothelioma attributable to occupational asbestos exposure was 83.2% and 38.4%, respectively, for men and women.[18] A case–control study by Rake et al.[19] of 622 diffuse malignant mesothelioma patients in the British population reported an attributable risk to asbestos of 86% in men and 38% in women; however, the authors pointed out that the cumulative female diffuse malignant mesothelioma death rate by age 70 is more than three times higher in the UK (0.037%) than in the United States (0.012%), suggesting that more than two-thirds of diffuse malignant mesotheliomas in British women born since the 1930s are caused by asbestos. This is more than the study suggested (38%) and would imply that at least 30% of female cases in the UK are caused either by environmental asbestos exposure or by occasional or ambient exposure in occupational settings.

The background rate has been estimated at between 1 and 4 cases per million persons per year.[17,20,21] In a review of 80 childhood cases, with an age range between 1 and 19 years, 67.5% were pleural, 25% peritoneal, and 7.5% pericardial.[5] Price and Ware[21] note that for most women, exposure sources for asbestos exposure would have been from use of asbestos-containing products in the home, general environmental exposure, and paraoccupational from other household members who worked in industries where there was asbestos exposure. As a group, women in the United States would have experienced increasing exposure due to the increase in asbestos consumption; however, there appeared to be no increased diffuse malignant mesothelioma incidence in women following the increased exposure according to the age-adjusted SEER data.[22] Therefore, the increased exposures were below a practical threshold for diffuse malignant mesothelioma.

There is case-study evidence that indicates that peritoneal diffuse malignant mesothelioma in women is very infrequently related to asbestos exposure and that it shows features that are different to those occurring in men, for example, relatively long survival periods.[23,24]

CONCLUSION

The majority of cases of pleural diffuse malignant mesothelioma in men are caused by exposure to amphibole asbestos. For peritoneal diffuse malignant mesothelioma, the epidemiologic evidence correlating time trends, incidence in both genders, and asbestos exposure suggests that most peritoneal diffuse malignant mesotheliomas are unrelated to asbestos exposure. The background lifetime probability of pleural and peritoneal diffuse malignant mesothelioma combined is estimated to be 3 to 4 per 10,000 individuals.[23,25] It is estimated that some 20% to 40% of all diffuse malignant mesotheliomas in the United States are now best regarded as idiopathic.

References

1. Wagner JC, Sleggs CA, Marchand P. Diffuse pleural mesothelioma and asbestos exposure in the North Western Cape Province. *Br J Ind Med* 1960;17:260–271.
2. Mark EJ, Yokoi T. Absence of evidence for a significant background incidence of diffuse malignant mesothelioma apart from asbestos exposure. *Ann NY Acad Sci* 1991;643:196–200.

3. Gibbs AR, Jones JS, Pooley FD, et al. Non-occupation malignant mesotheliomas. *IARC Sci Publ* 1989;90:219–228.
4. Roggli VL, Sharma A, Butnor KJ, et al. Malignant mesothelioma and occupational exposure to asbestos: a clinicopathologic correlation of 1445 cases. *Ultrastruct Pathol* 2002:26;55–65.
5. Fraire AE, Cooper S, Greenberg SD, et al. Mesothelioma of childhood. *Cancer* 1988;62:838–847.
6. Wagner E. Das tuberkelahnliche lymphadenom. *Arch Heilk* 1870;11:495–525.
7. Ilgren EB, Wagner JC. Background incidence of mesothelioma: animal and human evidence. *Regul Toxicol Pharmacol* 1991;13:133–149.
8. Ratzer ER, Pool JL, Melamed MR. Pleural mesotheliomas: clinical experiences with 37 patients. *Am J Radiol* 1967;99:863–880.
9. Borow M, Conston A, Livornes L, et al. Mesothelioma following exposure to asbestos: a review of 72 cases. *Chest* 1973;64:641–646.
10. Cochrane JC, Webster I. Mesothelioma in relation to asbestos fibre exposure: a review of 70 serial cases. *S Afr Med J* 1978;54:279–281.
11. Tagnon I, Blot WJ, Stroube RB, et al. Mesothelioma associated with the shipbuilding industry in coastal Virginia. *Cancer Res* 1980;40:3875–3879.
12. Oels HC, Harrison EG, Carr DT, et al. Diffuse malignant mesothelioma of the pleura: a review of 37 cases. *Chest* 1971;60:564–570.
13. Brenner J, Sordillo PP, Magill GB, et al. Malignant mesothelioma of the pleura: review of 123 patients. *Cancer* 1982;49:2431–2435.
14. Newhouse ML, Thompson H. Mesothelioma of pleura and peritoneum following exposure to asbestos in the London area. *Br J Ind Med* 1965;22:261–269.
15. Peto J, Henderson BE, Pike MC. Trends in mesothelioma in the United States, and the forecast epidemic due to asbestos during World War II. In: Peto R, Schneiderman M, eds., *Quantification of Occupational Cancer. Banbury Report 9*. New York, NY: Cold Spring Harbor Laboratory 1981:51–69.
16. McDonald AD, McDonald JC. Malignant mesothelioma in North America. *Cancer* 1980;46: 1650–1656.
17. Spirtas R, Heineman EF, Bernstein L, et al. Malignant mesothelioma: attributable risk of asbestos exposure. *Occup Environ Med* 1986;9:397–407.
18. Goldberg M, Imbernon E, Rolland P, et al. The French National Mesothelioma Surveillance Program. *Occup Environ Med* 2006;63:390–395.
19. Rake C, Gillam C, Hatch J, et al. Occupational, domestic and environmental mesothelioma risks in the British population: a case-control study. *Br J Cancer* 2009;100:1175–1183.
20. McDonald AD, McDonald JC. Malignant mesothelioma in North America. *Cancer* 1980;46: 1650–1656.
21. Price B, Ware A. Mesothelioma trends in the United States; an update based on surveillance, epidemiology and end-results program data for 1973 through 2003. *Am J Epidemiol* 2004;159: 107–112.
22. Price B, Ware A. Time trend of mesothelioma in the United States and projection of future cases: an update based on SEER data for 1973 through 2005. *Crit Rev Toxicol* 2009;39:576–588.
23. Kerrigan S, Turnnir R, Clement P, et al. Diffuse malignant epithelial mesotheliomas of the peritoneum in women. A clinicopathological study of 25 patients. *Cancer* 2002;94:378–385.
24. Weill H, Hughes JM, Churg A. Changing trends in U.S. mesothelioma incidence. *Occup Environ Med* 2004;61:438–441.
25. Moolgavkar SH, Meza R, Turim J. Pleural and peritoneal mesotheliomas in SEER: age effects and temporal trends, 1973–2005. *Cancer Causes Control* 2009;20:935–944.

SV40 Virus, Vaccines, and Disease

7

Richard L. Attanoos

Simian virus 40 (SV40) is a DNA polyoma virus that is found in monkeys and is a frequent contaminant of the rhesus macaque monkey kidney cell cultures used to grow vaccines.[1,2] The virus was introduced into the human population between 1955 and 1963 when it infected the Salk and Sabin polio and adenovirus vaccines. Accordingly, it is claimed that approximately 20 million persons received contaminated vaccines with live SV40.[3] SV40 has been associated with tumor development in animals and may be detected in various human neoplasms including diffuse malignant mesothelioma.[4,5] Medical and scientific opinion is divided in accepting a causal role for SV40 in the development of human tumors. This chapter presents a scientific review of the case *for* (Table 7-1) and *against* (Table 7-2) a carcinogenic role of SV40 in human cancer, and specifically diffuse malignant mesothelioma, by evaluation of in vitro, in vivo, and human studies.

Proponents of the view that SV40 causes diffuse malignant mesothelioma in human beings assert that SV40 could play a direct role in the carcinogenesis of human neoplasia. In diffuse malignant mesothelioma, this oncogenic activity could act in concert with asbestos.

Proponents of the view that SV40 does not cause human diffuse malignant mesothelioma assert that even if SV40 DNA sequences are present in diffuse malignant mesothelioma in human beings, there is no proof of anything more than spatial association, that is, the presence of an oncogenic virus in a tumor cell is not proof that it caused the cancer.

THE EVIDENCE *FOR* SV40 CAUSING HUMAN DIFFUSE MALIGNANT MESOTHELIOMA

SV40 Infection and Cell Transformation

The issue of whether SV40 may induce cancers in humans is controversial. SV40 exerts different effects in different cells dependent upon whether they are permissive, nonpermissive, or semipermissive.[6] In the natural host the cells are permissive, and virus-infected monkey cells are lysed. In nonpermissive rodent cells, SV40 causes cell transformation and division, but the infected cells cannot support viral replication. Accordingly the cell progeny reverts to a normal phenotype over time. In human cell cultures the cells are semipermissive indicating that they can be transformed and support low-level viral replication. Malignant transformation can only manifest if SV40 is integrated into the host genome. When SV40 infects human mesothelial cells, there is limited replication and limited cell death. The expression of SV40 tumor antigens (large T and small t antigens) in 100% infected cells leads to a high transformation rate (1 in 1,000 cells) (Fig. 7-1).

Table 7-1 The evidence *for* SV40 causing human tumors

- In vitro studies have demonstrated that SV40 induces cellular transformation in human cells. SV40 is a transforming virus.
- In vivo inoculation studies have demonstrated that SV40 could produce tumors (sarcomas, ependymomas, lymphomas, and diffuse malignant mesotheliomas) in hamsters.
- SV40 has been detected in human tumors in over 40 laboratories; many link SV40 to diffuse malignant mesothelioma or other tumors, which have been reported to be induced by SV40 in animals.
- SV40–transformed cell inoculates can induce tumors in human beings.

SV40 Oncogenesis

The capacity for SV40 to induce cell transformation is a function of its tumor antigen large T antigen.[7] This is a 90-kDa protein present in the nuclei of infected and transformed cells. Small t antigen is a 19-kDa protein detected in the cytoplasm of infected and transformed cells. Small t antigen has the capacity to increase the production of large T antigen and to potentiate its transforming ability, in part by inactivating p53.[8] SV40 large T antigen binds to various suppressor genes p53, Rb, and p107. SV40 inactivates p53, the Rb family, p107, p130, and RASSF1A.[9] SV40 induces telomerase activity, met, notch 1, and IGF-1R activation at the cell membrane. The activation of these oncogenes and growth factors subsequently activates the ERK-kinase pathway and AP 1 activity induces cell division. It has been proposed that because asbestos produces EGF receptor activation and AP 1 activity, the effects of SV40 large T antigen and asbestos act in concert in the induction of diffuse malignant mesothelioma.[10]

SV40 is implicated in loss of control of cell proliferation, increased cell division, and enhanced cell survival. The proponents of SV40 carcinogenesis point to the now growing evidence that it is a pathogen and that the weight of evidence extends beyond the arguments that SV40 is a carrier when detected in certain tumors and tissues.

SV40 Specificity

SV40 DNA sequences have been identified in pleural diffuse malignant mesothelioma, osteosarcoma, ependymoma and choroid plexus tumors, and various non-Hodgkin lymphomas.[11–15] Conversely, it has been demonstrated that SV40 is not present in stromal fibroblasts. This is demonstrable by various techniques including immunohistochemistry, in situ hybridization, and in situ polymerase chain reaction. This is significant as contamination cannot produce this finding. Over 40 different laboratories have detected SV40 DNA sequences in

Table 7-2 The evidence *against* SV40 causing human tumors

- There is an inconstant association between the detection of SV40 and diffuse malignant mesothelioma according to the International SV40 Working Group findings.
- SV40 is detectable in normal and neoplastic tissue with comparable frequency in some studies.
- No epidemiologic association between SV40 and diffuse malignant mesothelioma in human beings has been reported.

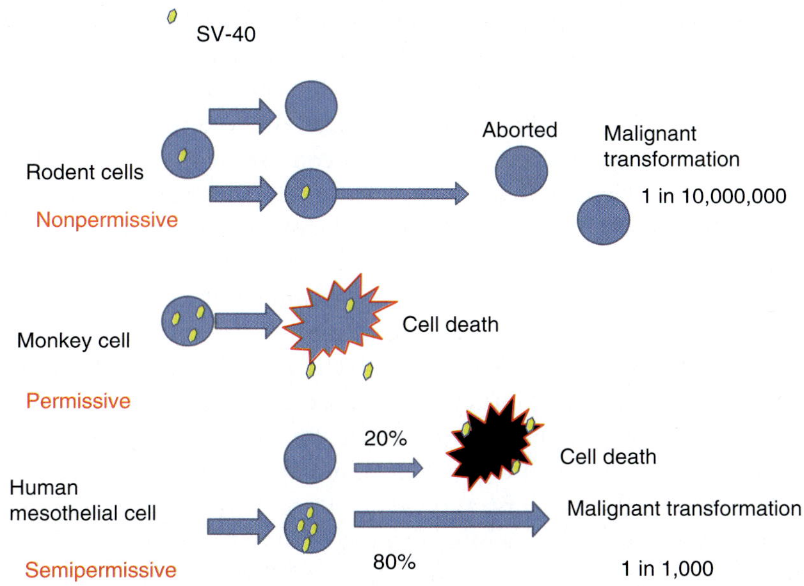

FIGURE 7-1: SV40 infection outcomes in nonpermissive, permissive, and semipermissive hosts.

select tumors on average 50% cases. Electron microscopy has also demonstrated virions in positive cases.

Geographic variations exist with negative results obtained in similar tumor cases from Austria, Turkey, and Finland where SV40–contaminated polio vaccines were not used. The proponents link the association with causative effect.

In human volunteers, SV40–transformed human cells induced subcutaneous tumors indicating that SV40 was capable of transforming human cells and capable of tumor induction in humans.[16]

THE EVIDENCE *AGAINST* SV40 CAUSING HUMAN DIFFUSE MALIGNANT MESOTHELIOMA

Some investigators have consistently failed to detect SV40–like sequences in diffuse malignant mesothelioma.[17,18] The most consistent criticisms of PCR technology are contamination and sensitivity. The proponents of the opposing viewpoints have utilized these factors to seek to undermine the validity of the opponents' supportive literature. False negatives have also been attributed to analytical failures as well as low sensitivity. In 1997, the International SV40 Working Group was established to standardize these analytical variations and address the issues of interlaboratory variations.[19] The National Cancer Institute funded nine laboratories to analyze blinded samples for SV40. Each laboratory received 25 paired duplicate samples of human diffuse malignant mesothelioma, a single set of 25 normal lung samples, as well as positive and negative control samples. The results showed that none of the diffuse malignant mesothelioma samples was consistently positive for SV40. Also, some researchers have found conflicting results on same tissue samples after analytical methodologic changes (with a false-negative initial result corrected on reanalysis).

To date, there is no epidemiologic evidence to support the view that there is an increased cancer risk in persons exposed to contaminated vaccines. In 1963, Fraumeni examined cancer mortality rates in persons <25 years old, within 4 years of the onset of the immunization program.[20] No mortality changes were detected for connective tissue, kidney, and brain tumors. The study results were limited given the short latent period from vaccine administration and follow-up. In 1970, Fraumeni reanalyzed the data in a smaller population of only children aged 6 to 8 years old in 1955, again concluding that there was no evidence of cancer increase in vaccinated children.[21] Cancer rates were higher in states within the United States receiving contaminated vaccines, but before and after vaccine administration. Further follow-up of neonates inoculated in the first week of life found no increase in cancer mortality after 20 years.[22] In 1998, Strickler et al.[23] examined the incidence of specific cancers reported to have contained SV40 DNA in a retrospective cohort study incorporating data from the Surveillance, Epidemiology and End Results (SEER) Program; the Connecticut Tumor Registry; and the National Mortality Statistics, overall approximately 10% of the population of the United States. The authors found that after 30 years of follow-up, there was no associated significant increase in diffuse malignant mesothelioma, osteosarcoma, or ependymoma incidence, despite the administration of SV40–contaminated vaccines. These results have been subject to substantial criticism, however, because there was a lack of age correlation and potential misapplication of statistical data. In 1999, Fisher et al.[24] examined trends in cancer incidence and the occurrence of specific tumors linked to SV40 over the 20-year period (1973 to 1993) using the SEER data. They found increases in age-adjusted incidence rates for all sites combined. The incidence was increased for diffuse malignant mesothelioma (90%), ependymoma (25%), and bone tumors (23%), although osteosarcomas remained stable with a slight increase of only 2.4%. Overall, the findings did not reach statistical significance for any tumor. In a Swedish study of cancer incidence over 1960 to 1990, of children inoculated with SV40–contaminated polio vaccine from 1957, found no increase in diffuse malignant mesothelioma or ependymoma (although other brain tumors were increased).[25] Danish epidemiologic study of those persons exposed to SV40–contaminated vaccine showed that they had a lower overall cancer risk than those not exposed and there was no increased incidence of mesothelioma, ependymoma, osteosarcoma, or non-Hodgkin lymphoma compared to those not exposed to virus.[26]

CONCLUSION

The scientific evidence presently indicates that there is insufficient basis to conclude that SV40 alone is capable of inducing diffuse malignant mesothelioma in human beings. However, it is reasonably plausible to conclude that SV40 may act in concert with asbestos in the development of diffuse malignant mesothelioma. The detection of SV40 in tumors does not demonstrate a causal relationship. Some researchers argue that SV40 may be an innocent passenger virus, and this is supported by the epidemiologic evidence, which has failed to identify an increase in those select tumors (known to have detectable quantities of SV40). However, it is of note that these epidemiologic studies are flawed because infected from noninfected cohorts are unknown. Further investigations are required to evaluate the cancer incidence in larger age-matched samples to facilitate an adequate statistical power to the study. Studies specific to diffuse malignant mesothelioma are confounded because of the rarity of the tumor, difficulty in diagnosis, and imprecision in risk estimates. Because there is a close association between the vast majority of diffuse malignant mesotheliomas and amphibole asbestos exposure, determining the isolated effect of SV40 in the causation of the tumor may be extremely problematic for many decades.

References

1. Sweet BH, Hilleman MR. The vacuolating virus, SV40. *Proc Soc Exp Biol Med* 1960;105:420–427.
2. Eddy BE, Borman GS, Grubbs GE, et al. Identification of the oncogenic substance in rhesus monkey kidney cell cultures as simian virus 40. *Virology* 1962;17:65–75.
3. Shah K, Nathanson N. Human exposure to SV40: review and comment. *Am J Epidemiol* 1976;103: 1–12.
4. Gerber P, Kirschstein RL. SV40 induced ependymomas in newborn hamsters. *Virology* 1962;18: 582–588.
5. Carbone M, Pass HI, Rizzo P. Simian virus 40 like DNA sequences in human pleural mesothelioma. *Oncogene* 1994;9:1781–1790.
6. Carbone M, Rizzo P, Pass HI. Simian virus 40, polio vaccines, and human tumours; a review of recent developments. *Oncogene* 1997;15:1877–1888.
7. Simmons DT. Transformation of polyoma viruses. In: Barbanti-Brodano G, Bendinelli M, Frieman H, eds., *DNA Tumors Viruses Oncogenic Mechanisms.* New York, NY: Plenum Publishing Company; 1995:27–50.
8. Tieman F, Zerrhan J, Deppert W. Cooperation of simian virus 40 large and small T antigens in metabolic stabilization in tumour suppressor p53 during cellular transformation. *J Virol* 1995;69:6115–6121.
9. Lill NH, Tevethia MJ, Eckner R, et al. P300 family members associate with the carboxyl terminus of SV40 large tumour antigen. *J Virol* 1997;71:129–137.
10. Carbone M, Pass HI, Mielel L, et al. New developments about the association of SV40 with human mesothelioma. *Oncogene* 2003;22:5173–5180.
11. Carbone M, Rizzo P, Procopio A, et al. SV40 like sequences in human bone tumors. *Oncogene* 1996;13:527–535.
12. Cristaudo A, Vivaldi A, Sensales G, et al. Molecular biology studies on mesothelioma tumor samples: preliminary data on H-ras, p21 and SV40. *J Environ Pathol Toxicol Oncol* 1996;14:29–43.
13. Testa JR, Carbone M, Hirvonen A, et al. A multi-institutional study confirms the presence and expression of simian virus 40 in human malignant mesothelioma. *Cancer Res* 1998;58:4505–4509.
14. Galateau Salle F, Bidet P, Iwatsubo Y, et al. SV40 like DNA sequences in pleural mesothelioma, bronchopulmonary carcinoma and non-malignant pulmonary diseases. *J Pathol* 1998;184: 252–257.
15. De Luca A, Baldi A, Esposito V, et al. The retinoblastoma gene family pRb/p105, p107, pRb2/p130 and simian virus 40 large T antigen in human mesotheliomas. *Nat Med* 1997;3:913–916.
16. Jensen F, Koprowski H, Pagano JS, et al. Autologous and homologous implantation of human cells transformed in vitro by SV40. *J Natl Cancer Inst* 1964;32:917–925.
17. Strickler HD, Goedert JJ, Fleming M, et al. Simian virus 40 and pleural mesothelioma in humans. *Cancer Epidemiol Biomarkers* 1996;5:473–475.
18. Krainer M, Schenk T, Zielinski CC, et al. Failure to confirm presence of SV40 sequences in human tumors. *Eur J Cancer* 1995;31A:1893.
19. The International SV40 Working Group. A multicenter evaluation of assays for detection of SV40 DNA and results in masked mesothelioma specimens. *Cancer Epidemiol Biomarkers Prev* 2001;10(5):523–532.
20. Fraumeni JF, Ederer F, Miller RW. An evaluation of the carcinogenicity of simian virus 40 in man. *JAMA* 1963;185:713–718.
21. Fraumeni JF, Stark CF, Gold E, et al. Simian virus 40 in poliovaccine: follow up of newborn recipients. *Science* 1970;167:59–60.
22. Mortimer EA Jr, Lepow ML, Gold E, et al. Long term follow-up of persons inadvertently inoculated with SV40 as neonates. *N Engl J Med* 1981;305:1517–1518.
23. Strickler HD, Rosenberg PS, Devesa GG, et al. Contamination of polio virus vaccines with simian virus 40 (1955–1963) and subsequence cancer rates. *JAMA* 1998;279:292–295.

24. Fisher SG, Weber L, Carbone M. Cancer risk associated with simian virus 40 contaminated polio vaccine. *Anti Cancer Res* 1999;19:2173–2180.
25. Olin P, Giesecke J. Potential exposure to SV40 in polio vaccines used in Sweden during 1957—no impact on cancer incidence rates 1960–1993. *Dev Biol Stand* 1998;94:227–233.
26. Engels EA, Katki HA, Nielsen NM, et al. Cancer incidence in Denmark following exposure to polio virus vaccine contaminated with simian virus 40. *J Natl Cancer Inst* 2003;95:24.

Medicolegal Considerations

8

▶ Timothy Craig Allen
▶ Richard L. Attanoos

The diagnosis of diffuse malignant mesothelioma in Western countries almost always sets into motion some form of legal process. The diagnosing pathologist must understand the potential pressures that may come to bear at the time of diagnosis, and resist them. In some cases, attorneys become involved merely at the suggestion that a patient may have diffuse malignant mesothelioma, and before a final diagnosis is rendered. Whether there is early attorney involvement or not, patients and their families, when faced with a pleural effusion or thickening for which diffuse malignant mesothelioma is in the differential, may lobby for the diagnosis. In some cases, the patient's surgeon or other treating physician may be swayed into pressuring the pathologist to render a diagnosis of diffuse malignant mesothelioma. Diffuse malignant mesothelioma is rare, and its possibility often causes an air of inappropriate excitement, to which even the unwary pathologist may be victim.

In any situation where diffuse malignant mesothelioma is in the differential diagnosis, the pathologist must be wary of such outside pressures and scrupulously avoid them. In the vast majority of cases, presentations for which diffuse malignant mesothelioma is in the differential ultimately are diagnosed as metastatic malignancies or fibrous pleuritis. The pathologist must recognize the rarity of the diagnosis of diffuse malignant mesothelioma, understand what is required for an accurate diagnosis, and proceed to final diagnosis in an efficient but unhurried and unbiased manner as one would in any diagnosis. In all but the most straightforward cases, consultation with a pulmonary pathologist with expertise in mesothelioma diagnosis is prudent.

As the diagnosis of diffuse malignant mesothelioma may take some time, it is important to make sure the surgeon and other treating physicians are aware of the case's status, so that the patient and family can be reassured that all is being done to obtain an accurate diagnosis.

Once a lawsuit involving diffuse malignant mesothelioma proceeds, it is unlikely that the diagnosing pathologist will be involved, as any arguments over the accuracy of the diagnosis will occur among pulmonary pathology expert witnesses. Nonetheless, the original diagnosing pathologist can perform an important service to society by working up any pleural case fully, clearly documenting the findings, whether it leads to the diagnosis of diffuse malignant mesothelioma or some other neoplastic or nonneoplastic pleural process that mimics diffuse malignant mesothelioma (Figs. 8-1 to 8-8). Seeking appropriate expert consultation at the time of original diagnosis is also of benefit. Indeed, in all cases of pleural lesions for which diffuse malignant mesothelioma is in the differential, a clear surgical pathology report can help lead to early dismissal of a case if the diagnosis is not diffuse malignant mesothelioma and can help lead to early settlement in cases of straightforward diffuse malignant mesothelioma. Whatever the diagnosis, society benefits by obtaining reduced litigation costs and a speedier litigation process.

Even in problematic cases, a well-sampled lesion, with appropriate immunostaining, and a clearly worded pathology report can make it possible for the pulmonary pathologist's expert witness to provide a strong expert opinion, again helping to dispose of the lawsuit in an efficient and cost-saving manner.

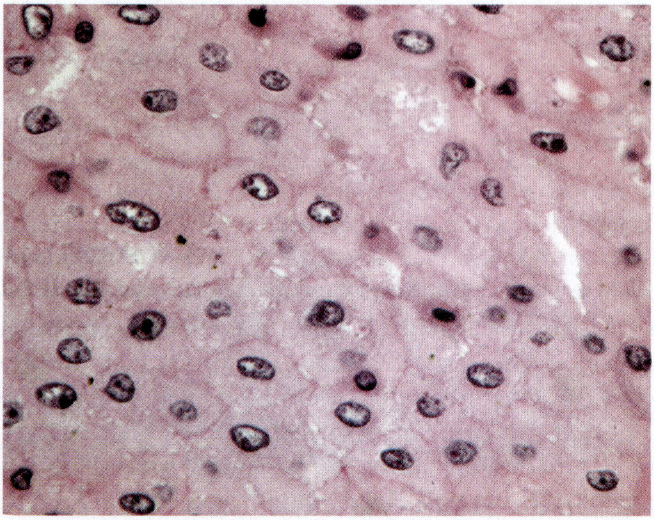

FIGURE 8-1: Deciduoid diffuse malignant mesothelioma; compare with Figure 8-2.

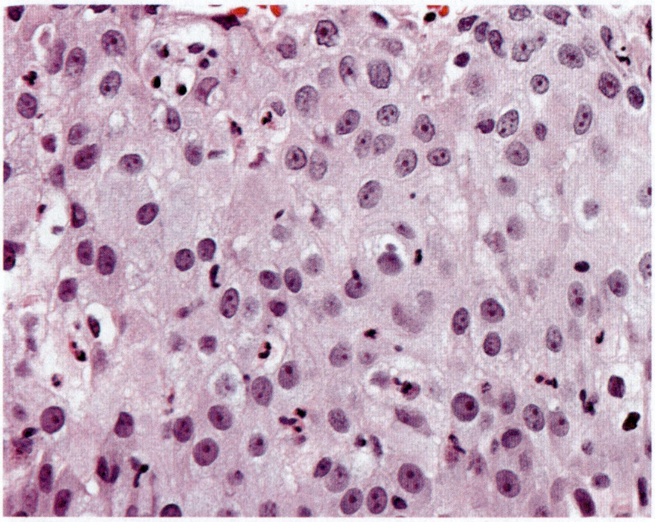

FIGURE 8-2: Squamous cell carcinoma metastatic to the pleura; compare with Figure 8-1.

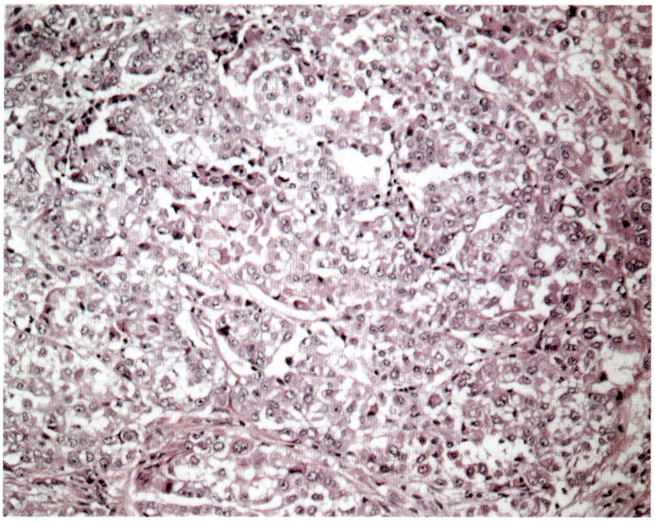

FIGURE 8-3: Clear cell pattern of diffuse malignant mesothelioma; compare with Figure 8-4.

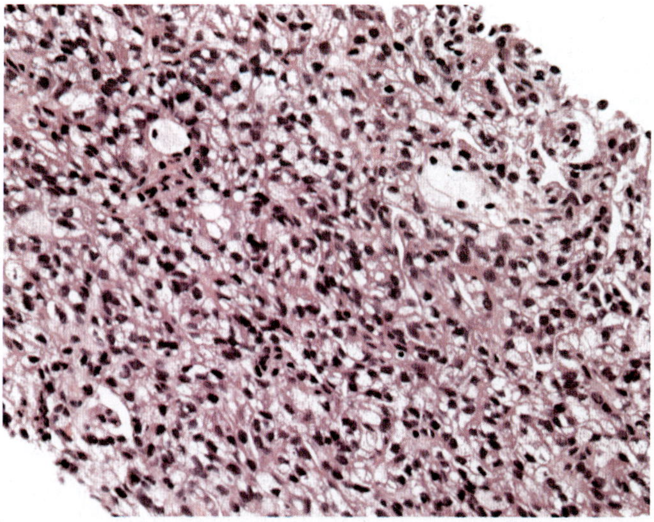

FIGURE 8-4: Renal cell carcinoma metastatic to the pleura; compare with Figure 8-3.

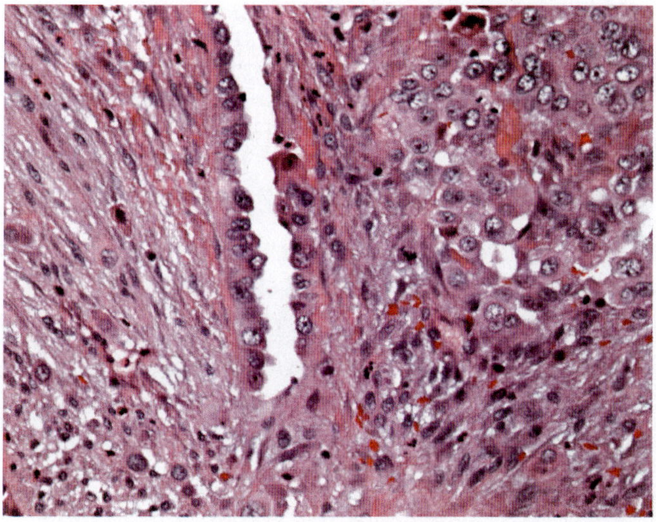

FIGURE 8-5: Biphasic diffuse malignant mesothelioma; compare with Figure 8-6.

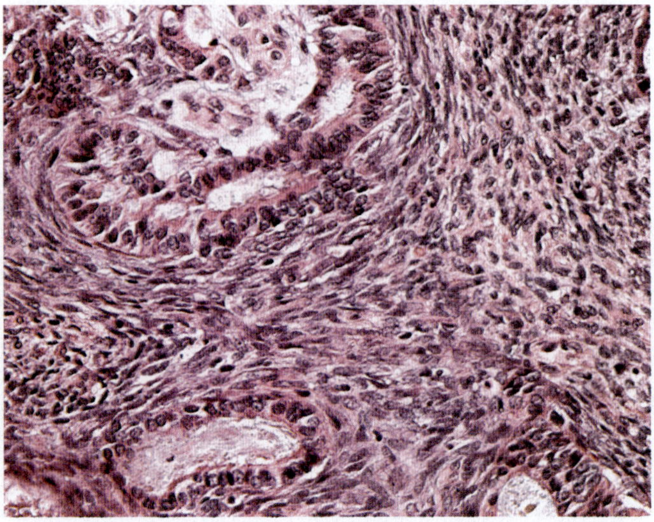

FIGURE 8-6: Pleural synovial sarcoma; compare with Figure 8.5.

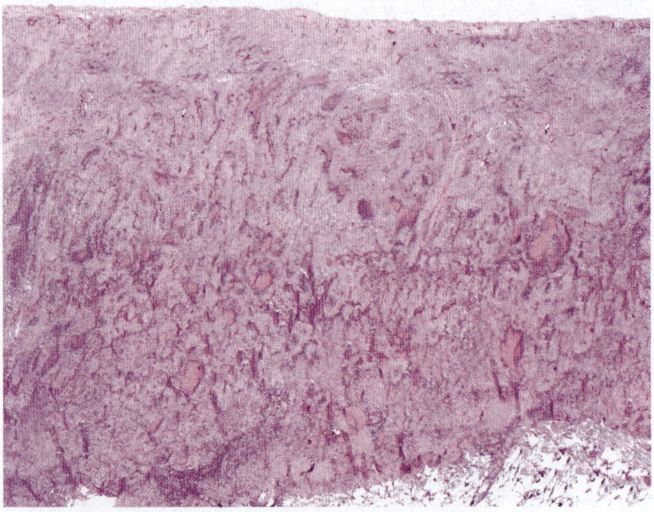

FIGURE 8-7: Epithelioid diffuse malignant mesothelioma; compare with Figure 8-8.

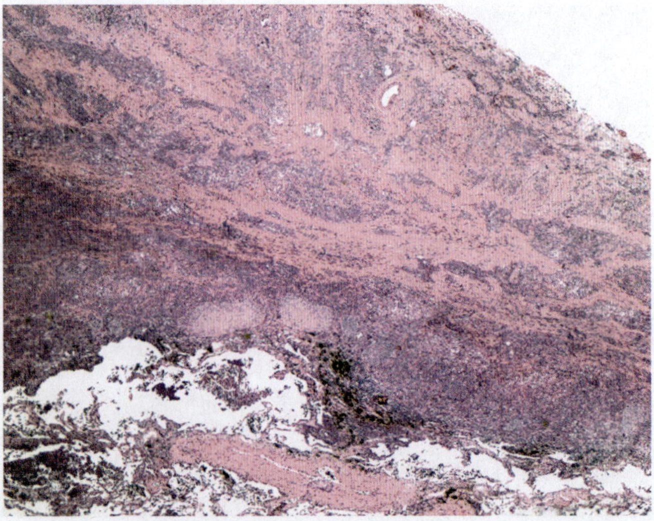

FIGURE 8-8: Pseudomesotheliomatous adenocarcinoma, lung primary; compare with Figure 8-7.

SECTION

II

Histopathology

Approach to the Serosal Biopsy

9

Richard L. Attanoos

A serosal biopsy may be deemed *adequate* when a good sample of mesothelium is present. This is more likely to be the case when open, laparoscopic, thoracoscopic, or radiologically guided biopsies are performed. The resting mesothelium is usually an attenuated layer of cuboidal cells (Fig. 9-1). A significant proportion of blind needle biopsies of the pleura contain muscle and fat without any mesothelium, and these should be reported as unsatisfactory. Generally, as with all branches of histopathology, the larger and more targeted the biopsy, the more likely one is to establish a correct and definitive diagnosis. In one comparative analysis of varied antemortem biopsy techniques in 45 subsequent autopsy-proven cases of diffuse malignant mesothelioma, needle biopsies were positive in only 16%, whereas open biopsies were positive in 95% to 100%.[1] In another series of 188 patients, needle biopsies provided a positive diagnostic yield in only 21%, whereas larger, thoracoscopic specimens gave a rate of 98%.[2] Biopsy size governs diagnostic yield and is itself dependent on underlying biopsy method and user technique and experience.

The most common artifacts observed in attempted pleural biopsies relate to crush effect or misappropriated tissue. The observation of a compressed eosinophilic membrane, derived from the skin epidermis, juxtaposed with underlying spindle cells may be misinterpreted as pleura rather than chest wall. The crushing of inflammatory cells may raise concerns of either metastatic small cell carcinoma or occult lymphoproliferative disease and prompt immunohistochemical evaluation.

After evaluating specimen adequacy, the next important consideration is to determine whether the biopsy shows definite malignancy or a reactive epithelioid, spindle cell proliferation or has mixed biphasic elements present (Fig. 9-2; Tables 9-1 to 9-3).

EPITHELIOID CELL PROLIFERATIONS

If a cellular epithelioid proliferation exists, it is important to establish its underlying nature: whether it is mesothelial, epithelial, or of another alternate histogenesis. Cytomorphologic features are useful in experienced hands to separate reactive epithelioid mesothelial cells from histiocytes, metastatic carcinoma, and other epithelioid malignancy; however, there are significant limitations on relying on morphologic characteristics alone because reactive mesothelial cells may demonstrate significant atypia and diffuse malignant mesotheliomas may exfoliate deceptively bland tumor cells. Considerable overlap exists (Figs. 9-3 and 9-4). Extreme caution should be exercised in diagnosing diffuse malignant mesothelioma on cytologic grounds alone, as exfoliative cytologic preparations do not allow for the evaluation of frank invasion, the only absolute criterion of malignancy. Indeed, diagnosing diffuse malignant

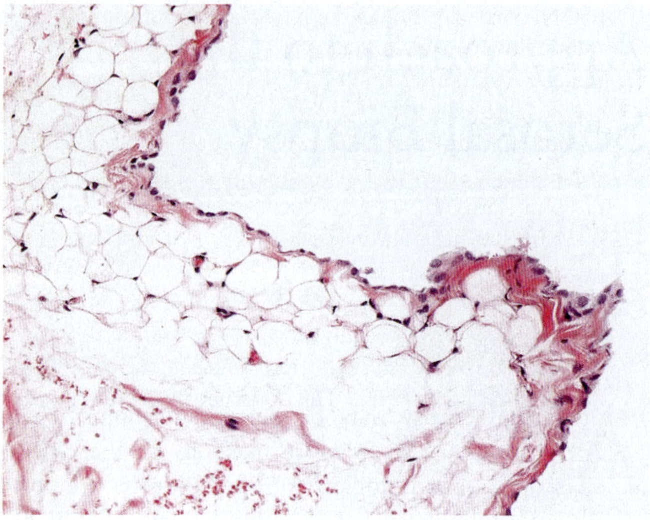

FIGURE 9-1: Resting mesothelium showing thin attenuated surface mesothelium on omental fat connective tissue.

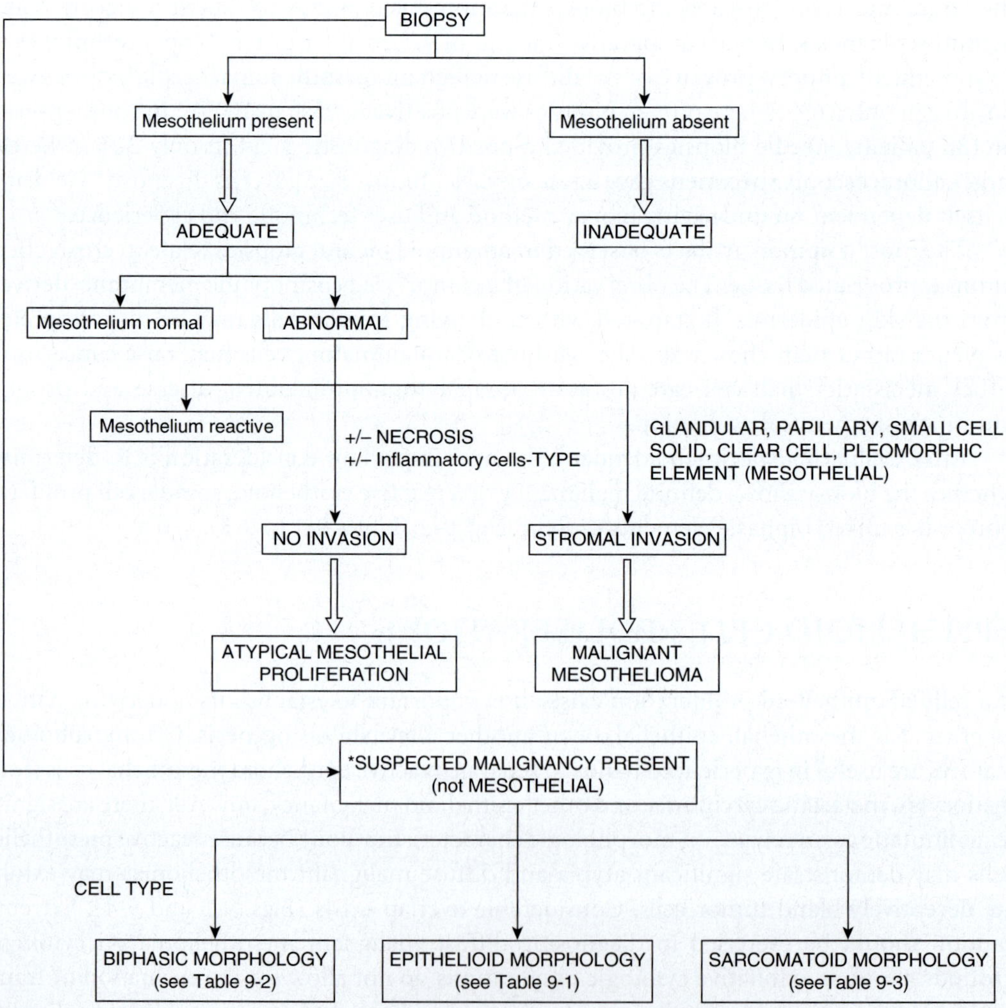

FIGURE 9-2: Approach to serosal biopsy interpretation.

Table 9-1 Diagnostic algorithm for epithelioid cell morphology

Mesothelioma	Differential Diagnosis

Glandular	Adenocarcinoma
	  Lung
	  Colon
	  Kidney
	  Ovary
	  Prostate
	Mesothelial hyperplasia

Solid epithelioid	Carcinoma Melanoma Germ cell neoplasia *Nodular mesothelial hyperplasia*
Small cell	Carcinoma Lymphoma Askin tumor Desmoplastic round cell tumor

Clear cell	Carcinoma
	  Kidney
	  Lung
	Melanoma (clear cell sarcoma)
	Germ cell neoplasia
	"Pecoma"

Lymphohistiocytoid	Lymphoepithelial carcinoma Thymic epithelial tumor Germ cell neoplasia Lymphoma *Inflammatory process*
Pleomorphic	Carcinoma Melanoma Sarcoma Lymphoma Germ cell neoplasia

mesothelioma on a cytologic specimen is essentially impossible and is not recommended. Additionally, sarcomatoid diffuse malignant mesotheliomas infrequently exfoliate diagnostic material, so in those cases a negative result holds no diagnostic weight. Immunohistochemistry has an important role in separating reactive from neoplastic mesothelial proliferations and determining underlying tumor histogenesis. Immunohistochemistry is reviewed in detail in Chapter 12.

The biopsy should ultimately be interpreted with knowledge of the clinical, radiologic, and direct observational findings of the sampling procedure (the thoracic and/or abdominal surgical opinion). This is most easily done through multidisciplinary meetings where the clinician, oncologist, surgeon, radiologist, and surgical pathologist are present. Diagnostic decision making will in part be impacted by knowledge of relevant concomitant medical conditions. In the pleura, for example, a patient may have had a pneumothorax,

Table 9-2 Diagnostic algorithm for biphasic morphology

Differential Diagnosis

Sarcomatoid carcinoma
  Lung
  Kidney

Carcinoma with desmoplastic stroma
Biphasic synovial sarcoma Epithelioid vascular sarcoma
Carcinosarcoma Malignant mixed mullerian tumor
Germ cell tumor
Cellular fibrous pleuritis and mesothelial hyperplasia

which could have resulted in a florid mesothelial proliferation in association with the features of a reactive eosinophilic pleuritis (Fig. 9-5). Distinction between reactive and malignant mesothelial proliferations is frequently problematic particularly in small biopsies. It should be borne in mind that both reactive and malignant mesothelial proliferations can be present simultaneously, for example, malignant mesothelioma may occasionally present with pneumothorax.[3] Eosinophil-rich infiltrates (seen commonly postpneumothorax) may be seen in certain drug reactions, in persons with autoimmune conditions, parasitic infestation, and certain rare hematolymphoid disorders (in particular myeloid leukemia, T-cell lymphoma, and Hodgkin lymphoma). Lymphoid-rich infiltrates may suggest tuberculosis and/or underlying lymphoproliferative disease. Formal hematopathologic referral should be initiated for accurate diagnosis, and this will be facilitated by multicolor immunofluorescence flow cytometric analysis, cytogenetic testing, as well as routine immunohistochemistry.

Table 9-3 Diagnostic algorithm for sarcomatoid morphology

Differential Diagnosis
Sarcomatoid carcinoma

Sarcoma
  Monophasic synovial sarcoma
  Solitary fibrous tumor
  Vascular sarcoma

Desmoid tumor
Melanoma
Cellular fibrous pleuritis
Retroperitoneal fibrosis

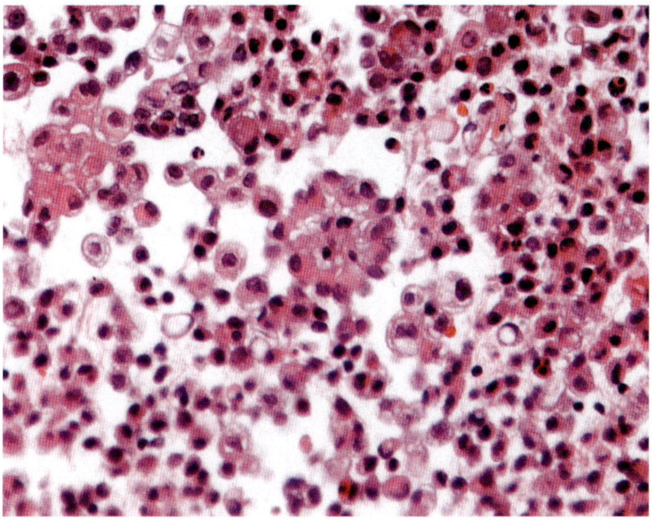

FIGURE 9-3: Epithelioid cells present as individual cells and morular clusters. Exfoliated mesothelial cells show intercellular "windows"; subsequent biopsies showed diffuse malignant mesothelioma.

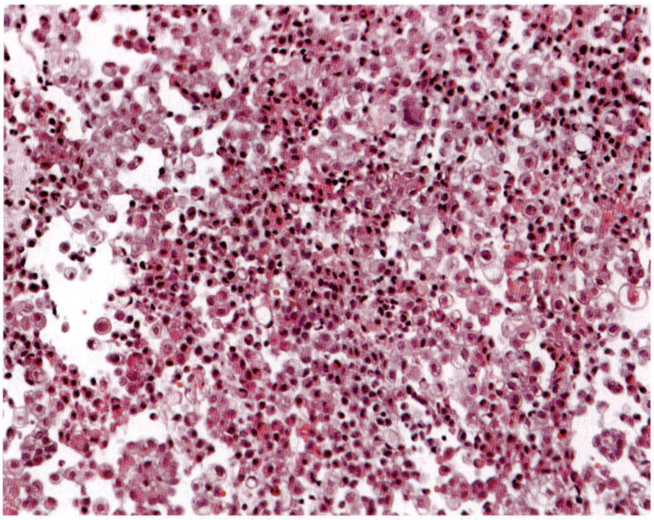

FIGURE 9-4: Cellular cytologic preparation showing sheets of dissociated epithelioid mesothelial cells. Subsequent diagnosis reactive hyperplasia.

Patients with collagen vascular disease may develop pleural effusion and exuberant mesothelial proliferations, with histiocyte and neutrophil-rich infiltrates and necrotic debris. The observation of necrosis, in particular, is worrisome of suspected underlying malignancy, but in subjects with rheumatoid nodules, necrosis may be seen and also in those with tuberculous pleurisy.

Large areas of necrosis may preclude a diagnosis of malignancy since there may be too few viable cells for the assessment of morphology or immunophenotype. However, necrosis within substantial areas of otherwise viable mesothelial cells raises the possibility of malignancy (albeit the stated caveats with tuberculosis, collagen vascular disease, etc.). Sometimes following prolonged surgery, acute inflammatory changes are seen within the pleura; these should not be interpreted as evidence of preexisting inflammation.

In the pleura and peritoneum, reactive mesothelial cell entrapment may be seen in persons with recurrent effusions of any causation on account of the successive cycles of inflammatory stimulation, mesothelial proliferation, and reparative fibrosis. In the peritoneum, marked reactive mesothelial cell entrapment may be seen in association with liver cirrhosis

FIGURE 9-5: Florid reactive mesothelial proliferation secondary to pneumothorax.

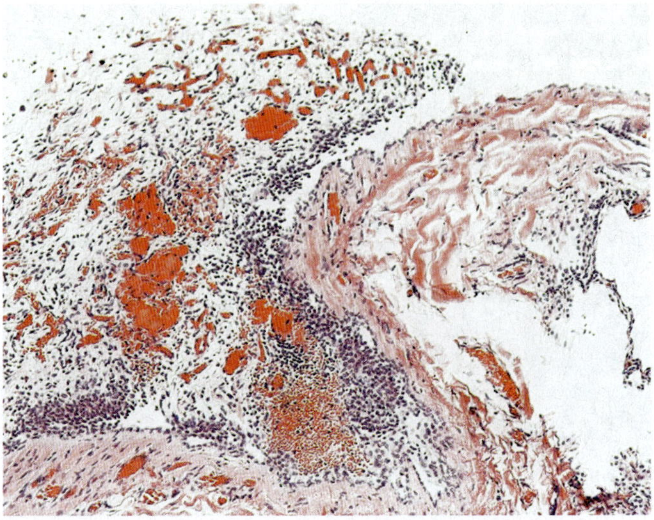

and ascites, endometriosis, and around omental–mesenteric decidual reactions.[4] Florid mesothelial proliferations can occur in hernia sacs (as so-called nodular histiocytic mesothelial hyperplasia) and in the pericardium.[5] On occasions these reactive mesothelial proliferations may exhibit marked atypia simulating malignancy. It is important to know whether clinically a diagnosis of diffuse malignant mesothelioma is seriously considered because a pathologist should be reluctant to make such a diagnosis if the clinician thinks the condition is more likely to be benign. Occasionally a pleural biopsy will be sectioned parallel to the pleural surface, which may give a mistaken impression of the mesothelial cells forming a solid tumor.

Diffuse malignant mesothelioma may involve lung and with intra-alveolar growth mimicking organizing pneumonia and desquamative interstitial pneumonia.[6] The morphologic features, which should be taken into account with respect to assessment of malignancy, include (1) extent and complexity of cellular proliferation, (2) cytologic atypia, (3) zonation, (4) presence and severity of inflammation, and (5) invasion.

Reactive mesothelial proliferations usually occur in parallel layers and sheets, whereas the presence of complex papillary structures in pleural biopsies points toward malignancy. Cytologic pleomorphism, mitoses, and inflammation are unreliable determinants of benign versus neoplastic mesothelial proliferation. Indeed, if there is severe inflammation evident, then associated mesothelial proliferations need to be interpreted with great caution. Diffuse malignant mesothelioma may be complicated by empyema, and the overlying inflammation may mask the presence of diffuse malignant mesothelioma. Unequivocal invasion of structures such as fat, chest wall muscle, or lung parenchyma allows for a confident diagnosis of malignancy to be made.

In serosal biopsies full-thickness mesothelial proliferations or stromal nodules are nearly always malignant, whereas mesothelial proliferations in the superficial cavity–associated regions may be benign or malignant (Fig. 9-6). Stromal invasion can be mimicked by entrapment of mesothelial cells within fibrous tissue in inflammatory processes, but these often have a linear arrangement, which parallels the surface. One needs to be aware that artifactual displacement of mesothelium in closed needle biopsies can occur.

Mesothelial cell inclusions in lymph nodes may mimic metastatic diffuse malignant mesothelioma but must be interpreted with caution. They are usually limited to the subcapsular sinus or show sinusoidal distribution without lymph node effacement. Immunohistochemistry is important in defining their benign nature.

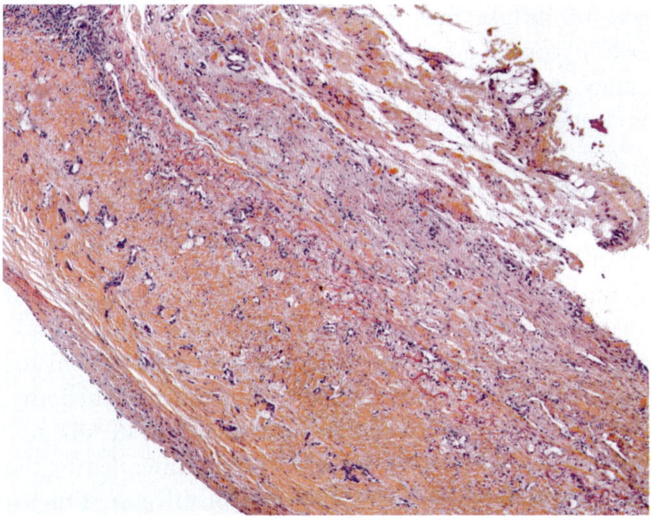

FIGURE 9-6: Frank invasion of pleura by malignant mesothelioma; the superficial aspect shows linearity mimicking benignancy/mesothelial entrapment (**upper left**), but deep invasion is present (**lower right**).

ALGORITHMIC APPROACH FOR EPITHELIOID TUMORS OF THE SEROSA

Distinguishing epithelioid diffuse malignant mesothelioma from various carcinomas and other epithelioid malignancies is facilitated by necessary ancillary testing. Epithelioid malignancies of the serosal tissues are generally either metastatic carcinomas or diffuse malignant mesothelioma. Both are cytokeratin positive. If a diffuse malignant mesothelioma has epithelioid morphology, it should be positive for both broad-spectrum cytokeratins and at least one of the commonly positive mesothelial markers (calretinin, cytokeratin 5/6, WT-1, D2-40). Accordingly, if a serosal-based epithelioid malignancy is negative particularly for varied tested cytokeratins, then diagnoses other than diffuse malignant mesothelioma or carcinoma should be seriously considered. These include malignant melanoma, malignant vascular sarcomas (low-grade epithelioid hemangioendothelioma or high-grade epithelioid angiosarcoma), primitive neuroectodermal tumor (Askin tumor), or some non-Hodgkin lymphomas (notably anaplastic large cell lymphoma) (Table 9-1).

Diffuse malignant mesothelioma may be subject to different morphologic patterns and subtypes in an individual tumor. For this reason there is merit in sampling the tumor widely, particularly when sarcomatoid elements of the tumor predominate (which do not readily allow for definitive diagnosis) and resection or necropsy material is available. It is recognized that the epithelioid component of diffuse malignant mesothelioma is more readily identifiable as such by immunohistochemical markers and other ancillary studies. For this reason, a careful search for epithelioid components is worthwhile, even if they represent a minority component of the tumor.

Searching for epithelioid elements in diffuse malignant mesothelioma may be problematic, but there should be focus on seeking out lymphatic tumor emboli as these often exhibit epithelioid morphology. Metastatic tumor in involved lymph nodes may provide suitable diagnostic tissue to run an immunohistochemical panel, alongside the main tumor. Extreme caution should be exercised in interpreting immunomarkers in areas of necrosis and where pleural diffuse malignant mesothelioma infiltrates lung parenchyma as there will inevitably be cell entrapment.

The morphologic variant forms of diffuse malignant mesothelioma do not have significant prognostic importance (except for the adverse prognosis of desmoplastic diffuse malignant mesothelioma). Instead, they provide the pathologist with an appreciation that diffuse malignant mesothelioma may generate a vast differential of histogenetically diverse tumors, most unrelated to asbestos.

The utility of these immunohistochemical panels is governed by tumor morphology, patient gender, and anatomic site of the neoplasm. In particular, in the female peritoneum, diffuse malignant mesothelioma should be distinguished from primary and secondary Mullerian neoplasms (predominantly serous carcinoma). This is not straightforward because of the common coelomic origin of the tumors and resultant similar morphologic and immunophenotypic characteristics, and it necessitates using a series of immunohistochemical markers to facilitate any suspected diagnosis of diffuse malignant mesothelioma. Incorporating a broad panel of immunomarkers is more reliable for accurate diagnosis than reliance on the morphologic tumor appearances alone. It is recommended by the International Mesothelioma Interest Group to incorporate at least two positive mesothelial markers and two positive epithelial markers together with a broad-spectrum cytokeratin.[7] Because of the commercial availability of antibodies, the individual choice of antibody will depend on personal preference and laboratory experience. Some markers have lower specificity and sensitivity than others, and the pathologist should always be mindful of potential false-positive and false-negative rates. The role of immunohistochemistry and molecular cytogenetic testing in the diagnosis of diffuse malignant mesothelioma and its mimics is detailed in other chapters.

ALGORITHMIC APPROACH FOR BIPHASIC AND SARCOMATOID TUMORS OF THE SEROSA

For serosal biphasic and sarcomatoid tumors, the differential diagnoses generally lie between diffuse malignant mesothelioma, sarcomatoid carcinoma, and sarcoma. Reactive conditions may mimic each morphologic type, most notably chronic fibrous pleuritis mimicking desmoplastic diffuse malignant mesothelioma. In certain anatomic sites and genders, specific tumors should be considered at an early stage. For example, in the female peritoneum, malignant mixed mullerian tumor (carcinosarcoma) and malignant teratomatous germ cell neoplasms are far more common than in the counterpart pleural site. Conversely biphasic and sarcomatoid diffuse malignant mesothelioma in the peritoneum is rare. Immunohistochemistry and molecular cytogenetic testing is potentially useful in evaluating these cases and discussed in other chapters (Tables 9-2 and 9-3).

THE UTILITY OF THE ASBESTOS EXPOSURE HISTORY IN EVALUATING SEROSAL BIOPSIES FOR SUSPECTED DIFFUSE MALIGNANT MESOTHELIOMA

Most diffuse malignant mesotheliomas are associated with prior asbestos exposure, and the strength of the association varies with anatomical tumor site, gender, and asbestos fiber type and industry.[8,9] Epidemiologic and mineralogic studies show that amphiboles cause the vast majority of diffuse malignant mesothelioma in men. Some authorities believe that virtually all diffuse malignant mesotheliomas are asbestos related.[10] Many experts believe that spontaneous or idiopathic mesotheliomas do occur, and highlight non–asbestos-related risk factors for the disease (such as environmental erionite exposure, radiation, and simian virus 40 inoculation).[11–13]

The background lifetime probability of pleural and peritoneal diffuse malignant mesothelioma combined is estimated to be 3 to 4 per 10,000 individuals.[9,14] For peritoneal diffuse malignant mesothelioma, the epidemiologic evidence correlating time trends, incidence in both genders, and asbestos exposure suggests that most peritoneal diffuse malignant mesotheliomas are potentially unrelated to asbestos.

Asbestos is undoubtedly associated with a lower percentage of peritoneal diffuse malignant mesotheliomas when compared to pleural counterpart tumors. Historically, peritoneal diffuse malignant mesotheliomas are typically associated with higher cumulative asbestos exposures and exposures to commercial amphiboles. There exists no robust epidemiologic link between peritoneal diffuse malignant mesothelioma and chrysotile exposure.

Because of the association between asbestos and diffuse malignant mesothelioma, it is not uncommon for pathologists to regard the subjects' asbestos exposure history as a criterion in ascertaining the diagnosis of diffuse malignant mesothelioma. It cannot be overstated that this is incorrect and flawed approach. The pathologic diagnosis of the tumor is based on the combination of the morphologic findings plus ancillary information such as mucin studies, immunohistochemistry, electron microscopy, and molecular analyses. In the presence of adequate pathologic tissue, the asbestos exposure history is irrelevant and should absolutely not be used to overturn an alternate diagnosis.

Only in the absence of diagnostic pathologic tissue can the asbestos exposure history be considered as a factor in the clinical diagnostic decision-making process. If a patient has a history of asbestos exposure and has imaging information, which demonstrates a diffuse pleural based tumor, then because diffuse malignant mesothelioma is the most common tumor to show this imaging feature, it becomes the "default" clinical diagnosis. This may prompt the physician to request a tissue diagnosis. The gold standard for the diagnosis of diffuse malignant mesothelioma is the tissue biopsy result. Cytologic specimens are limited and do not allow for a confident diagnosis. Accordingly, considerable caution should be exercised by the surgical pathologist; a misinterpreted case has far reaching medical and legal consequences.

In the peritoneum and other serosal sites, the approach is different because diffuse malignant mesothelioma is far less common than disseminated carcinomatosis (from the gastrointestinal tract, pancreas, or ovaries) and other tumors. For this reason, diffuse malignant mesothelioma is not the "default" diagnosis, and further investigations, preferably biopsy diagnosis, are necessary.

References

1. Attanoos RL, Gibbs AR. The comparative accuracy of different pleural biopsy techniques in the diagnosis of malignant mesothelioma. *Histopathology* 2008;53:340–344.
2. Boutin C, Rey F. Thoracoscopy in pleural malignant mesothelioma: a prospective study of 188 consecutive patients. *Cancer* 1993;72:389–393.
3. Sheard J, Taylor W, Soorae A, et al. Pneumothorax and mesothelioma in patients over the age of 40. *Thorax* 1991;46:584–585.

4. Clement PB. Endometriosis, lesions of the secondary Mullerian system and pelvic mesothelial proliferations. In: Kurman RJ, ed. *Blaustein's Pathology of the Female Genital Tract.* 5th ed. New York, NY: Springer Verlag; 2002:729–789.
5. Rosai J, Dehner LP. Nodular mesothelial hyperplasia in hernia sacs. A benign reactive condition stimulating a neoplastic process. *Cancer* 1975;35:165–172.
6. Nind N, Attanoos RL, Gibbs AR. Unusual intraparenchymal growth patterns of malignant pleural mesothelioma. *Histopathology* 2003,42:150–155.
7. Husain AN, Colby TV, Ordonez GN, et al. Guidelines for pathologic diagnosis of malignant mesothelioma: a consensus statement from the International Mesothelioma Interest Group. *Arch Pathol Lab Med* 2009;133(8):1317–1331.
8. Wagner JC, Sleggs CA, Marchand P. Diffuse pleural mesothelioma and asbestos exposure in the North Western Cape Province. *Br J Ind Med* 1960;17:260–271.
9. Price B, Ware A. Mesothelioma trends in the United States: an update based on surveillance, epidemiology, and end results program data for 1973 through 2003. *Am J Epidemiol* 2004;159:107–112.
10. Mark EJ, Yokoi T. Absence of evidence for a significant background incidence of diffuse malignant mesothelioma apart from asbestos exposure. In: Third wave of asbestos disease: Exposure to asbestos in place. Landrigan PJ, Kazemi H, eds. *Ann NY Acad Sci* 1991;643:196–213.
11. Selcuk ZT, Coplu I, Kalyoncu AF, et al. Malignant pleural mesothelioma due to environmental mineral fibre exposure in Turkey: analysis of 135 cases. *Chest* 1992;102:790–796.
12. Peterson JT, Greenberg SD, Buffler PA. Non asbestos-related malignant mesothelioma: a review. *Cancer* 1984;54:951–956.
13. Carbone M, Pass HI, Rizzo P, et al. Simian virus 40-like sequences in human pleural mesothelioma. *Oncogene* 1994;9:1781–1790.
14. Moolgavkar SH, Meza R, Turim J. Pleural and peritoneal mesotheliomas in SEER: age effects and temporal trends, 1973–2005. *Cancer Causes Control* 2009;20:935–944.

Morphologic Variants and Their Mimics

10

Richard L. Attanoos
Allen R. Gibbs

The 2004 World Health Organization Classification of Lung and Pleural tumors recognizes that diffuse malignant mesothelioma is separated into four histologic subtypes. However, within these subtypes there is a myriad of morphologic patterns, which can occur in a variety of combinations[1–3] (Table 10-1). This can result in significant diagnostic problems since a range of tumors can enter the differential diagnosis. In general, these morphologic variants have no significant prognostic importance, and all are associated with asbestos. Sometimes one pattern predominates, but at other times there may be a more even mixture.

DIFFUSE MALIGNANT MESOTHELIOMA

Epithelioid Diffuse Malignant Mesothelioma

The most frequent morphologic variants observed within the epithelioid subtype are tubulopapillary, adenomatoid (microcystic), and solid sheets. Other less frequent patterns include clear cell, deciduoid, pleomorphic, or poorly differentiated and small cell.[4–8] Some authors have also described low-grade myxoid-rich, signet ring cell, "mucin"-positive, glycogen-rich, lipoid cell, balloon cell, and Gaucher cell–like variants for descriptors of the tumor cells. The morphologic features of the individual tumor cells may show mild to marked atypia and varying degrees of mitotic activity. However, the tumor cells in the tubulopapillary and adenomatoid variants are typically bland with open nuclei, eosinophilic cytoplasm, and low mitotic rate. Psammoma bodies are observed in approximately 5% of the tubulopapillary variant cases. The tumor cells lining the tubules and papillae are cuboidal or low columnar in shape and form on fibrovascular connective tissue cores or as delicate epithelioid cell papillae devoid of stroma (Figs. 10-1 and 10-2). Mesothelial papillary proliferation is a useful morphologic predictor of diffuse malignant mesothelioma over benign mesothelial hyperplasia. On cross section, prominent collagen cores may be seen in diffuse malignant mesothelioma, a feature more commonly identified in cytologic preparations (Fig. 10-3).

The main differential diagnosis lies between epithelioid diffuse malignant mesothelioma and adenocarcinoma. For pleura diffuse malignant mesothelioma, the differential diagnosis is predominantly pulmonary adenocarcinoma that has either metastasized or spread directly to the pleura. For peritoneal diffuse malignant mesothelioma, the differential diagnoses include peritoneal carcinomatosis from the primary and secondary (female) mullerian system (particularly serous carcinoma), pancreas, and intestinal tract. Other differential diagnoses include well-differentiated papillary mesothelioma and adenomatoid tumor. Both

Table 10-1 Morphologic variants of diffuse malignant mesothelioma

<table>
<tr><th>Epithelioid</th><th>Sarcomatoid</th></tr>
<tr><td>Tubulopapillary</td><td>Not specified (MFH-like)</td></tr>
<tr><td>Microcystic</td><td>Desmoplastic</td></tr>
<tr><td>Solid</td><td>Leiomyoid</td></tr>
<tr><td>Small cell</td><td>Heterologous</td></tr>
<tr><td>Pleomorphic</td><td></td></tr>
<tr><td>Deciduoid</td><td></td></tr>
<tr><td>Clear cell</td><td></td></tr>
<tr><td>Myxoid rich</td><td></td></tr>
<tr><td>Signet ring cell</td><td></td></tr>
<tr><td colspan="2">Lymphohistiocytoid</td></tr>
<tr><td colspan="2">Transitional</td></tr>
</table>

MFH-like, Malignant fibrous histiocytoma–like.

of the latter neoplasms tend to be localized compared with the diffuse serosal growth pattern observed in diffuse malignant mesothelioma. Immunohistochemistry is useful in distinguishing diffuse malignant mesothelioma from adenocarcinoma (see Chapter 12) but has no utility in separating the different mesothelial tumors.

In the adenomatoid variant, the tumor forms microcystic areas or lace-like structures (Figs. 10-4 to 10-6). Secretory cell changes may be prominent imparting a signet ring cell morphology (Fig. 10-7). This is morphologically indistinguishable from signet ring cell (diffuse) adenocarcinoma. These features may mimic adenocarcinoma, adenoid cystic carcinoma, or vasoformative tumors. Immunohistochemistry allows for the distinction of the tumors by incorporating mesothelial, epithelial, and endothelial markers in the antibody panel.

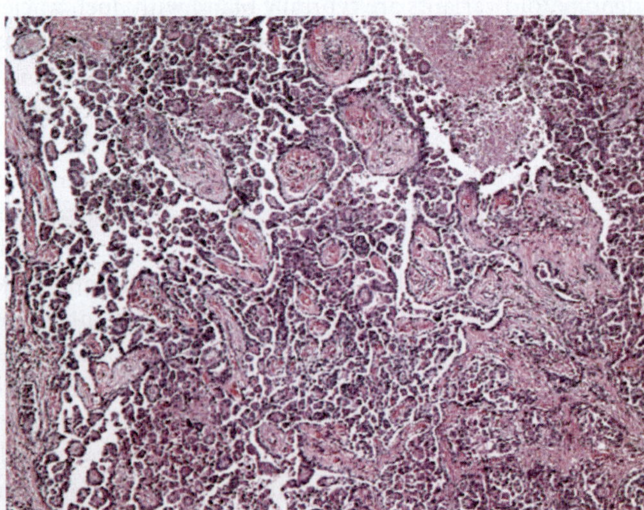

FIGURE 10-1: Diffuse malignant mesothelioma, epithelioid subtype. Low power showing tubulopapillary variant.

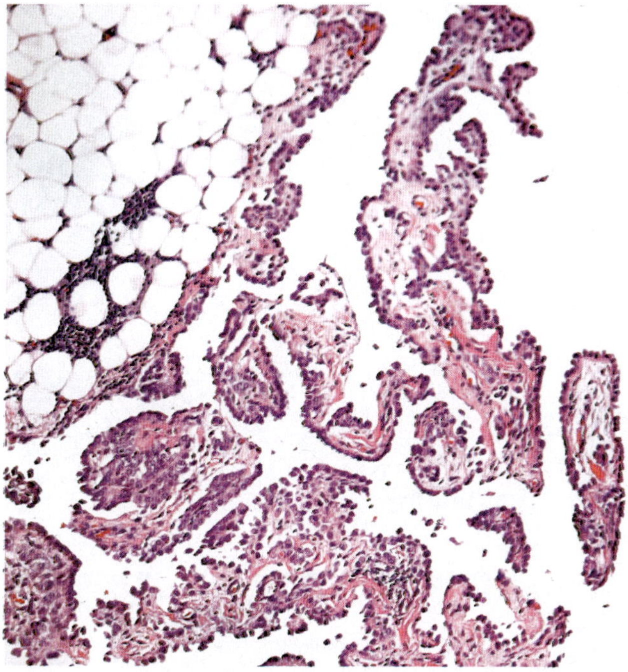

FIGURE 10-2: Diffuse malignant mesothelioma, epithelioid subtype; tubulopapillary variant.

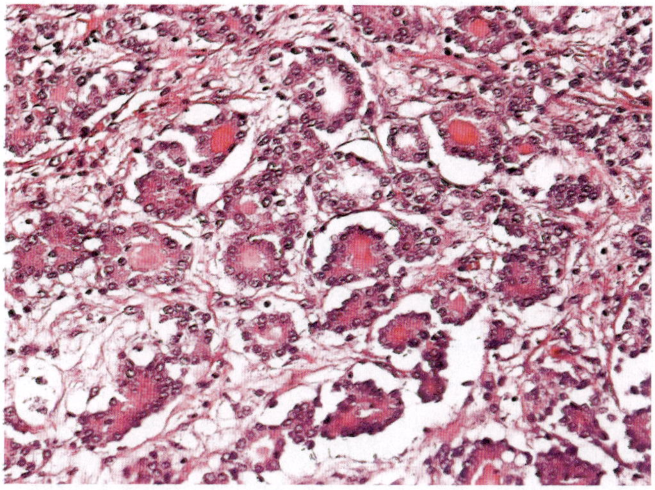

FIGURE 10-3: Diffuse malignant mesothelioma, epithelioid subtype. Higher power showing prominent hyaline collagen cores in the tubulopapillary variant.

The production of abundant extracellular mucins is common in the myxoid-rich variant of epithelioid diffuse malignant mesothelioma. Tumor cells are often seen "free floating" in myxohyaline matrix (Fig. 10-8). Sometimes there is dystrophic calcospherites present (Fig. 10-9). This pattern mimics colloid or mucinous adenocarcinoma. In the peritoneum, the accumulations of jelly-like mucosubstance mimic the clinical condition of pseudomyxoma peritonei most often associated with low-grade mucinous tumors of appendiceal origin following transmural invasion.

Epithelioid diffuse malignant mesothelioma with prominent intra- and extracellular accumulations of acid mucosubstance is occasionally able to produce an unusual tinctorial staining pattern with neutral mucin stains (mucicarmine- and diastase-pretreated periodic acid–Schiff) (Fig. 10-10). This has prompted some investigators to call the lesion

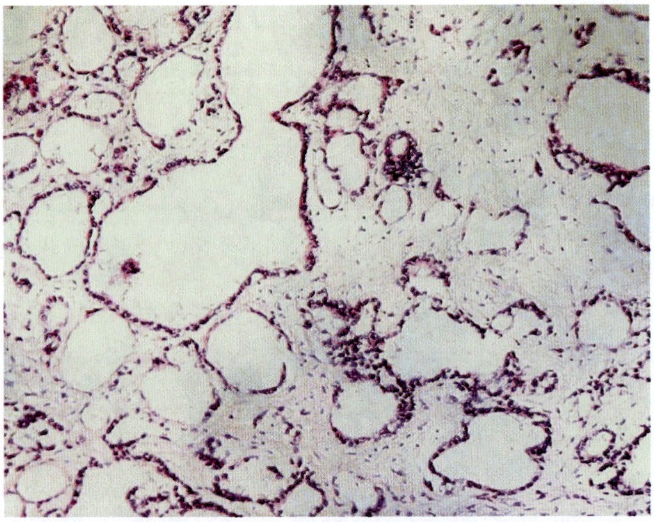

FIGURE 10-4: Diffuse malignant mesothelioma, epithelioid subtype. Adenomatoid variant with microcystic areas.

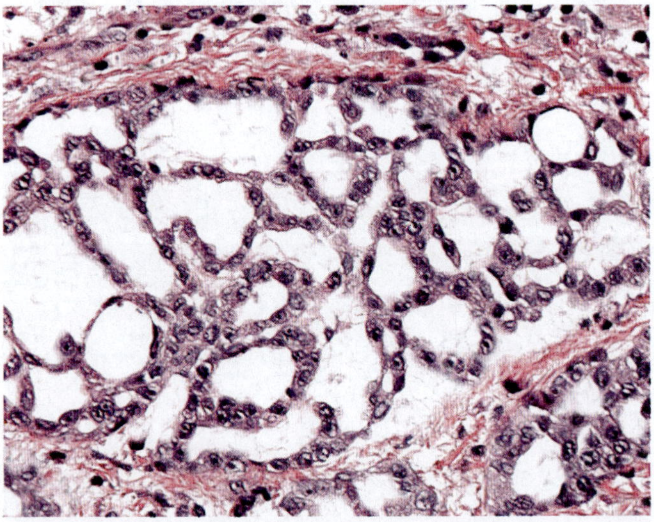

FIGURE 10-5: Diffuse malignant mesothelioma, epithelioid subtype. Higher power of adenomatoid variant.

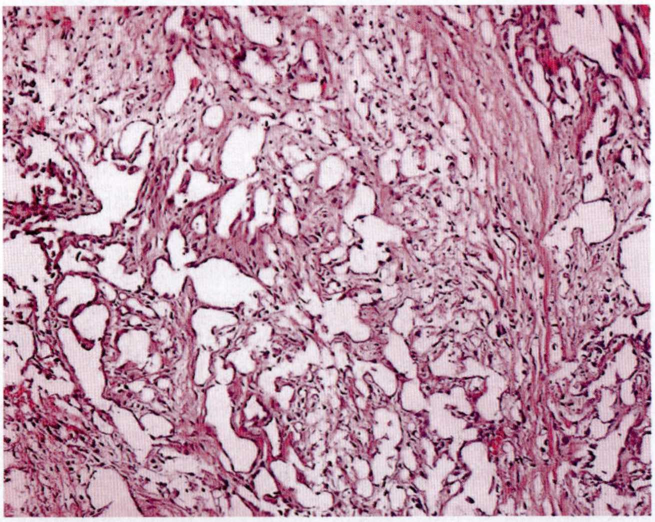

FIGURE 10-6: Diffuse malignant mesothelioma, epithelioid subtype. The adenomatoid variant here mimics a vasoformative neoplasm.

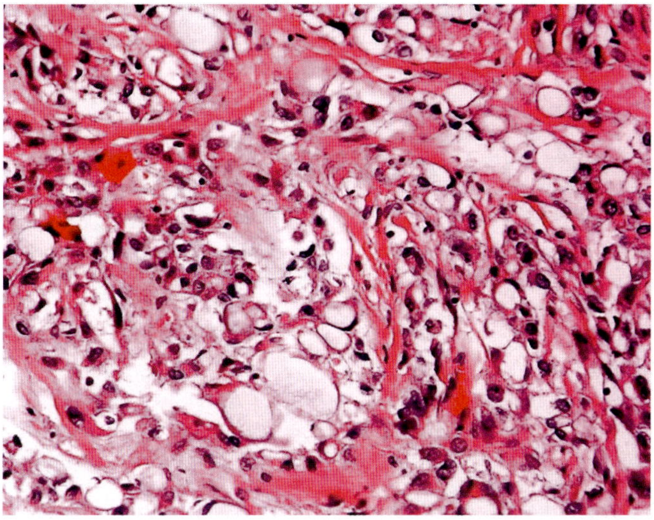

FIGURE 10-7: Diffuse malignant mesothelioma, epithelioid subtype. Prominent signet ring cell morphology mimicking diffuse adenocarcinoma.

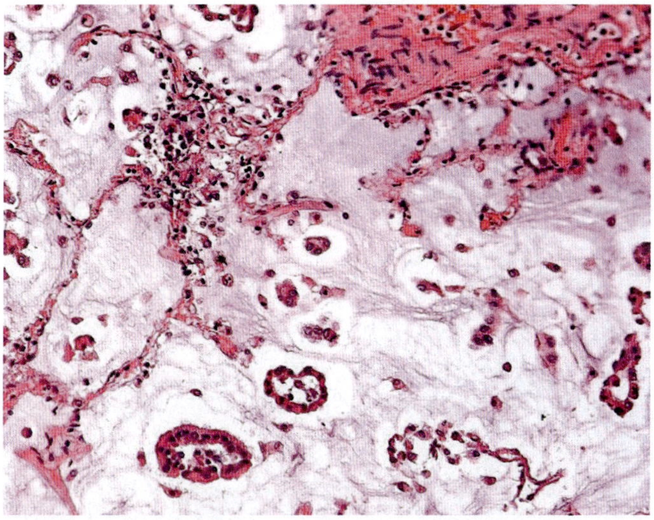

FIGURE 10-8: Diffuse malignant mesothelioma, epithelioid subtype. The myxoid-rich variant with abundant extracellular mucosubstance and free-floating tumor cells.

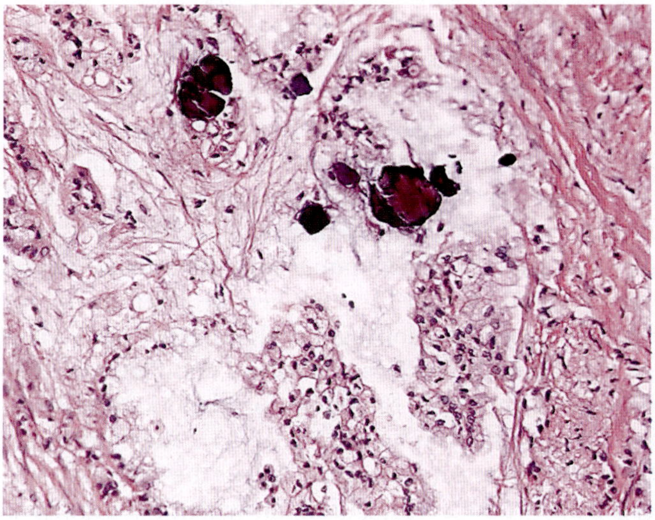

FIGURE 10-9: Diffuse malignant mesothelioma, myxoid variant with calcospherites present.

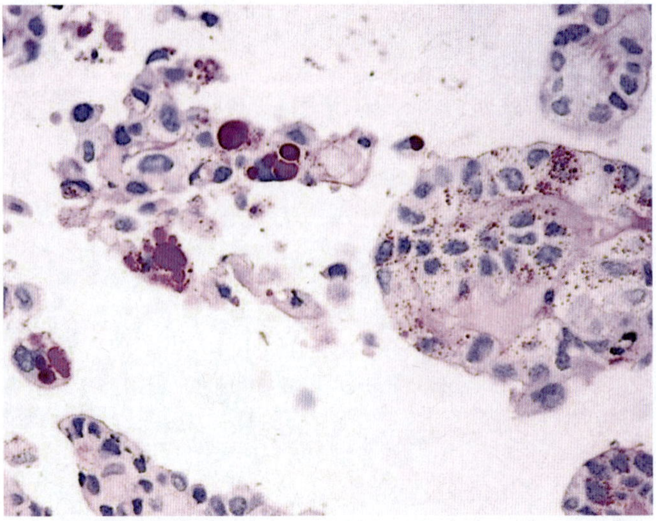

FIGURE 10-10: Diffuse malignant mesothelioma, so-called "mucin-positive" variant. Diastase-resistant periodic acid-schiff staining observed mimicing adenocarcinoma. (Reprinted from Shepherd NE, Warren BF, Williams GT, et al., eds. *Morson and Dawson's Gastrointestinal Pathology*. 5th ed. Oxford, UK: Wiley-Blackwell; 2013, with permission.)

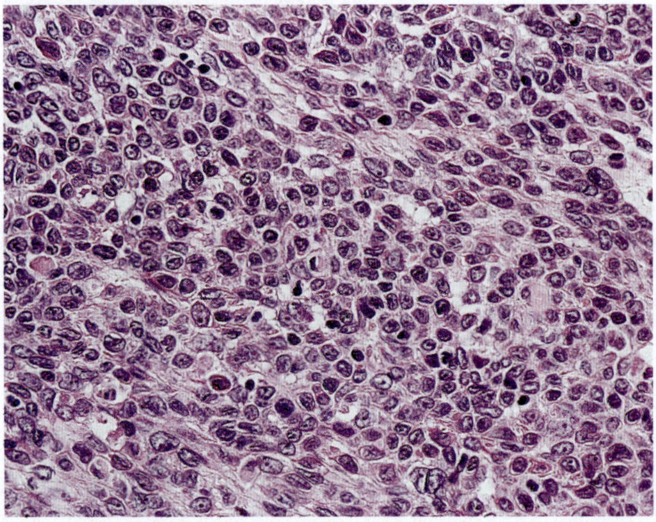

FIGURE 10-11: Diffuse malignant mesothelioma, epithelioid subtype, solid variant.

mucin-positive diffuse malignant mesothelioma. This highlights to the unwary pathologist that mucin histochemistry must be carefully interpreted. Indeed, the histochemical reaction may be abolished by pretreatment with hyaluronidase, and the reaction has been attributed to crystalline hyaluronate deposition. Some authors have reported aberrant immunohistochemical reactions with polyclonal CEA and Leu M1 (CD 15) in this variant of epithelioid diffuse mesothelioma; however, these have not been widely confirmed.

The solid variant contains large polygonal cells, which mimic large cell carcinoma, and some tumor giant cells may be present (Figs. 10-11 and 10-12). When the latter are prominent, the term pleomorphic diffuse malignant mesothelioma or poorly differentiated variant is used (Fig. 10-13), and the differential diagnosis includes that of any undifferentiated or anaplastic epithelioid malignancy—namely, anaplastic carcinoma, amelanotic melanoma, some epithelioid variant sarcomas, and anaplastic lymphoma (Fig. 10-14). The mitotic rate in these tumors is relatively high. It is important to emphasize that despite the close morphologic mimicry of these anaplastic epithelioid tumors, only diffuse malignant mesothelioma

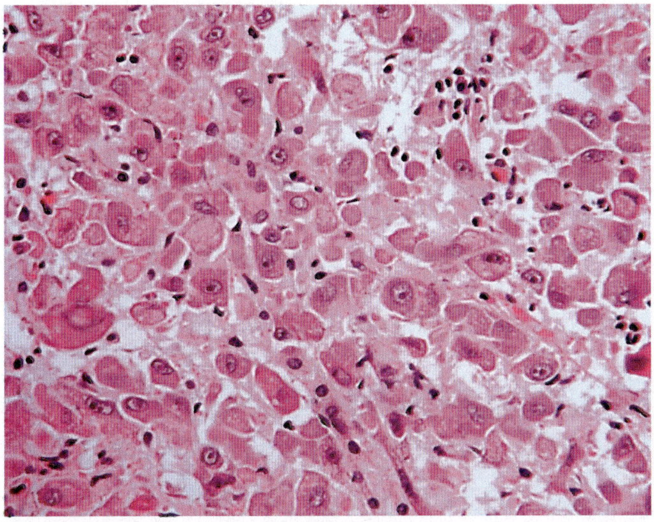

FIGURE 10-12: Diffuse malignant mesothelioma, epithelioid subtype, higher power of solid variant.

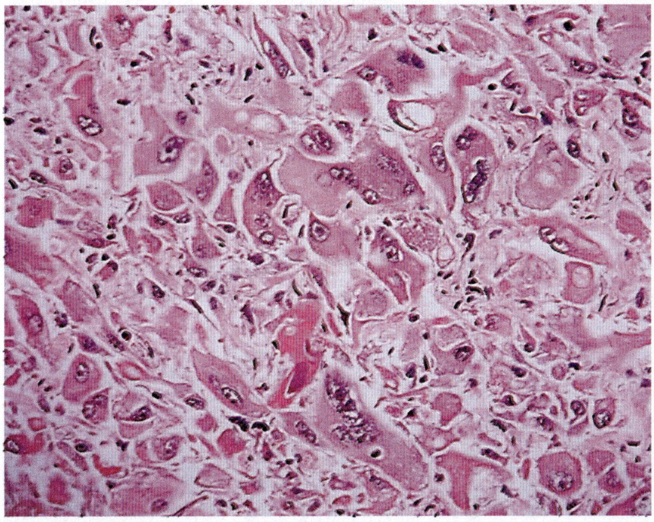

FIGURE 10-13: Diffuse malignant mesothelioma, epithelioid subtype, pleomorphic or poorly differentiated variant. Prominent polygonal epithelioid cells with numerous giant cells.

and bronchogenic carcinoma are asbestos-related neoplasms, and in each the causation issues are distinct and different. It is important to consider the anatomic distribution of the tumor as well as rely on ancillary marker studies.

The deciduoid form is composed of cells with plump eosinophilic cytoplasm similar to the deciduoid cells of the uterus seen in pregnancy. It has been proposed that this is a specific morphologic variant identified in young females, although subsequent authors have contested this and the author concurs with this latter position.[7,8] There is, in fact, a subjective arbitrary division between solid epithelioid, deciduoid, pleomorphic, and transitional diffuse malignant mesothelioma (Fig. 10-15), a term used for the designation of a morphologic variant with indistinct borderline features between epithelioid and sarcomatoid elements.

Epithelioid diffuse malignant mesothelioma may form sheets of clear tumor cells (Figs. 10-16 and 10-17). This is consequent to the accumulation of glycogen or acid mucins. There is a subjective overlap between clear cell diffuse malignant mesothelioma and the variants termed glycogen-rich, lipoid cell, balloon cell, and Gaucher cell–like types.[9,10] When clear

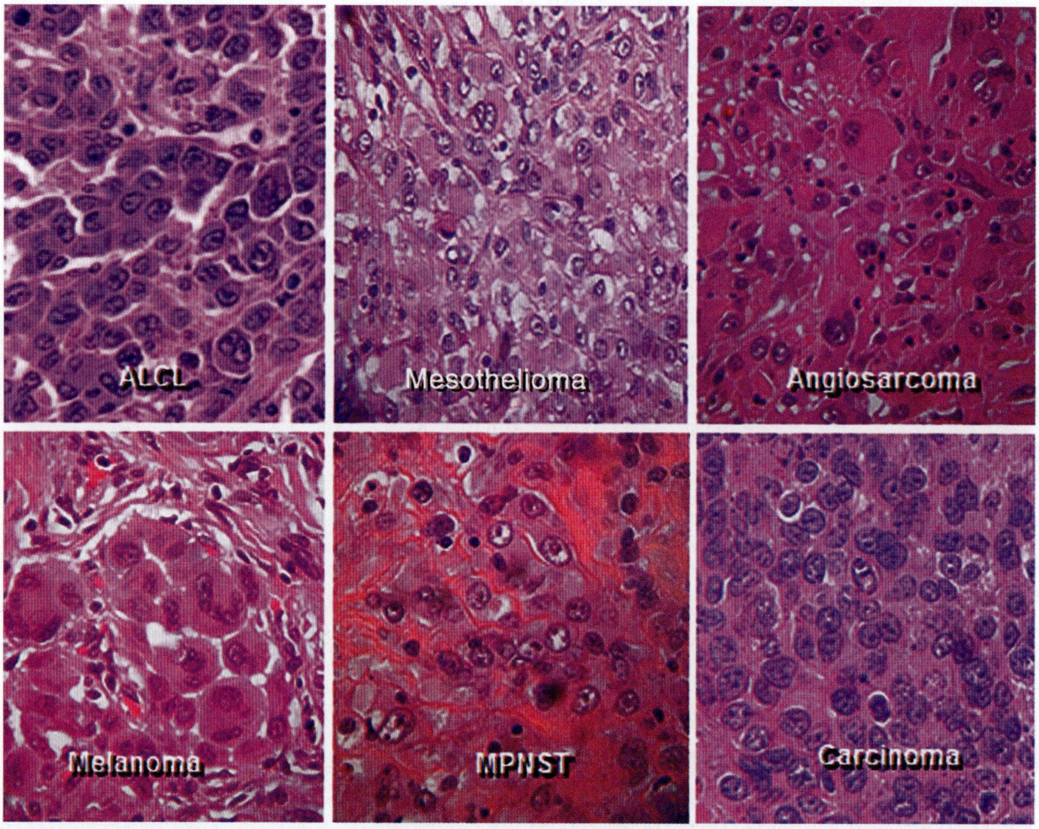

FIGURE 10-14: Diffuse malignant mesothelioma, solid epithelioid subtype mimicking various undifferentiated epithelioid tumors. (ALCL, anaplastic large cell lymphoma; MPNST, malignant peripheral nerve sheath tumor.)

FIGURE 10-15: Diffuse malignant mesothelioma, transitional variant. Most of the tumor cells are elongated and spindled, while a minority appears more polygonal and epithelioid.

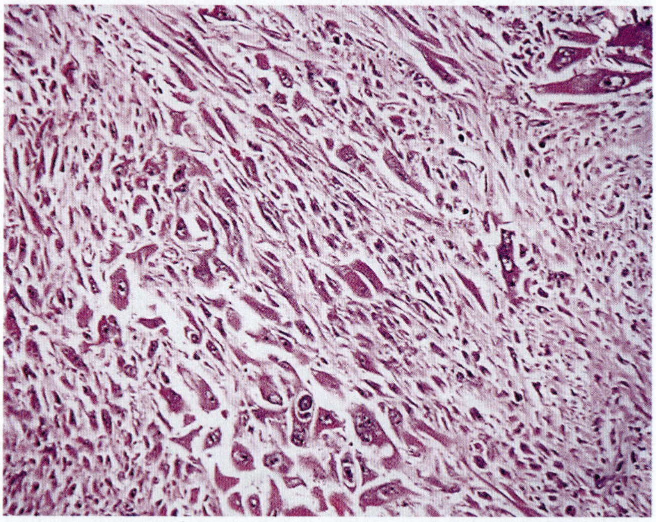

cells are prominent, metastatic renal cell carcinoma and clear cell carcinoma of the lung enter the differential diagnosis. Clinical factors are often useful in separating the tumors. Other clear cell tumors such as clear cell sarcoma (malignant melanoma of soft parts)[11] (Fig. 10-18) and perivascular epithelioid cell tumor (PEComa) should be considered if the initial immunohistochemistry is not definitive. Immunohistochemistry is useful in separating most epithelioid

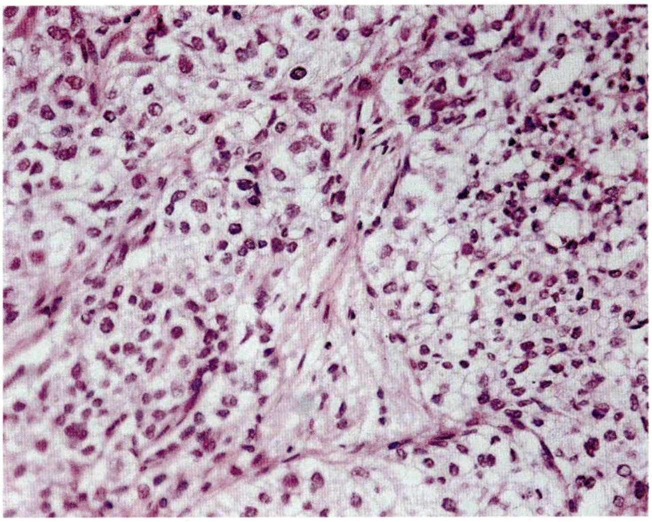

FIGURE 10-16: Diffuse malignant mesothelioma, epithelioid, clear cell variant.

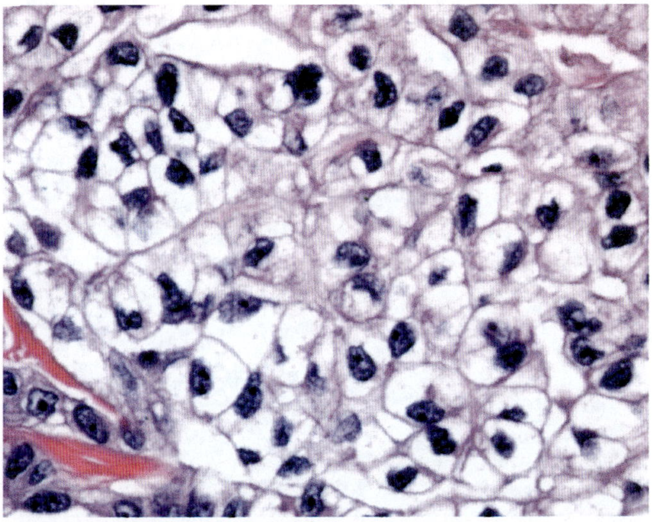

FIGURE 10-17: Diffuse malignant mesothelioma, epithelioid, clear cell variant, higher power.

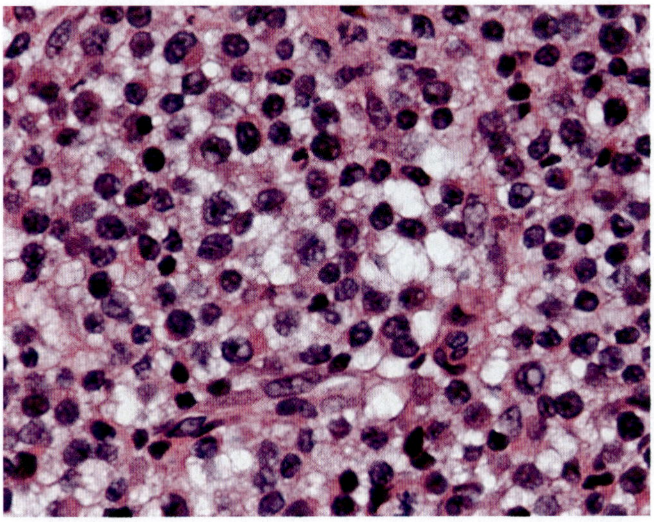

FIGURE 10-18: Clear cell sarcoma (malignant melanoma of soft parts) metastatic to the pleura mimicking clear cell diffuse malignant mesothelioma.

diffuse malignant mesotheliomas from metastatic renal cell carcinoma, but the latter is known to express epithelial and mesothelial markers reflecting the common embryonic ancestry, so pitfalls do exist. Molecular cytogenetics is useful in identifying clear cell sarcoma, with its distinct translocation of t(12; 22) (q13;q12) in approximately 75% cases.[12]

The small cell variant of diffuse malignant mesothelioma comprises sheets of small hyperchromatic cells with high nuclear to cytoplasmic ratio. Cellular cohesion is poor imparting an autolytic appearance (Fig. 10-19). Small cell diffuse malignant mesothelioma has to be distinguished primarily from small cell carcinoma of the lung, a number of non-Hodgkin lymphomas, and the rare desmoplastic small round cell tumor and Askin tumor (small round cell tumor of the thoracopulmonary region). Tumor rosettes, karyorrhexis, and hematoxyphilic staining of blood vessels typically seen in small cell carcinoma are absent in small cell diffuse malignant mesothelioma.[6] Desmoplastic small round cell tumor (Fig. 10-20) and Askin tumor may both closely mimic small cell diffuse malignant mesothelioma and have similar serosal distributions.[13] The Askin tumor has a distinct translocation

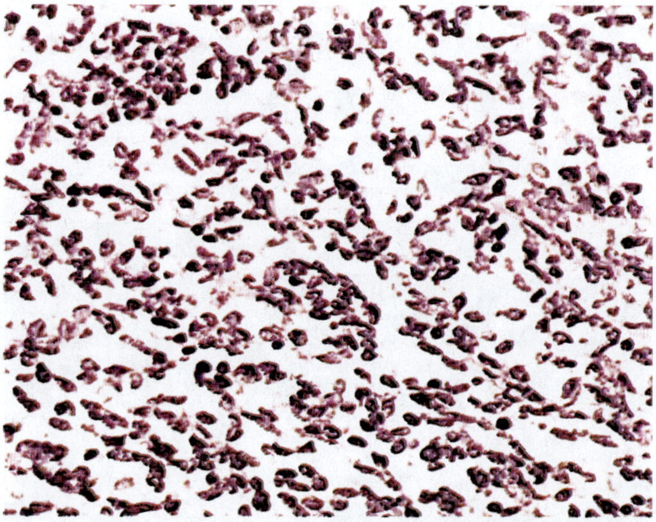

FIGURE 10-19: Diffuse malignant mesothelioma, small cell variant. Tumor cells show high nuclear to cytoplasmic ratio and discohesion mimicking small cell carcinoma.

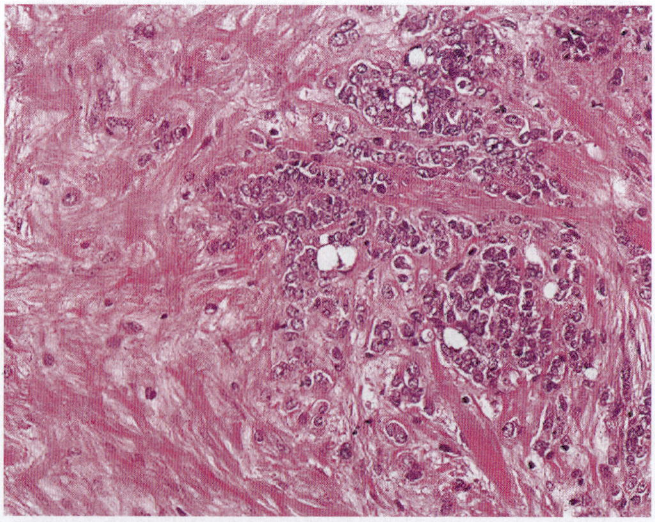

FIGURE 10-20: Desmoplastic small round cell tumor. The tumor cells are interspersed with a paucicellular desmoplastic stroma.

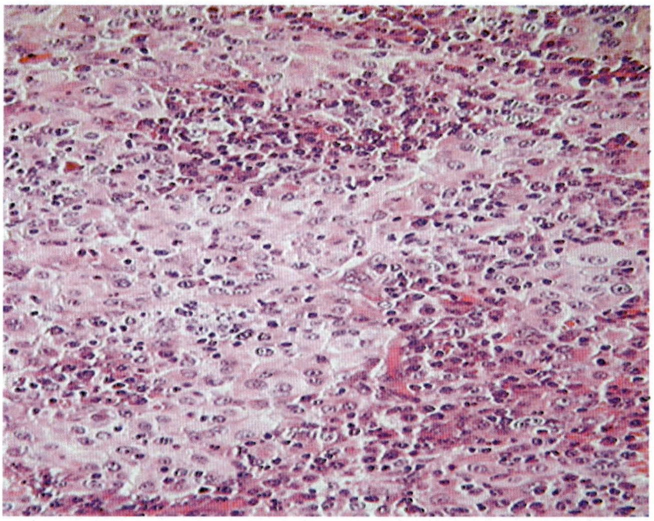

FIGURE 10-21: Diffuse malignant mesothelioma, epithelioid subtype, lymphohistiocytoid variant with numerous plasma cells.

(11;22) (q24; q12) observed in 80% cases, and the desmoplastic round cell tumor exhibits translocation (11;22)(p13;q12). Immunohistochemistry and cytogenetic analysis are effective in separating the tumors (see Chapters 12 and 18).

The lymphohistiocytoid variant constitutes <1% of diffuse malignant mesotheliomas. It was originally reported as a variant of sarcomatoid diffuse malignant mesothelioma, but epithelioid forms of the tumor have been observed also to have florid associated lymphoid and histiocytic infiltrations. The variant is usually composed sheets of epithelioid mesothelial cells set in a dense infiltrate of lymphocytes and plasma cells (Fig. 10-21). The tumor may mimic non-Hodgkin lymphoma, thymic epithelial tumor, germ cell neoplasia, or an inflammatory process, depending on the extent of the associated host response.[14] Careful use of immunohistochemistry will enable the correct diagnosis.

Sarcomatoid Diffuse Malignant Mesothelioma

Sarcomatoid diffuse malignant mesotheliomas occur primarily in the pleura, being rare in pure form in the peritoneum and tunica vaginalis testis. Indeed, pure sarcomatoid diffuse malignant mesotheliomas of the peritoneum comprised only 2% of 326 sarcomatoid diffuse malignant mesotheliomas in one study.[15] The primary differential diagnoses of spindle cell tumors of the pleura include sarcomatoid diffuse malignant mesothelioma, sarcomatoid carcinoma, and sarcoma. Sarcomatoid diffuse malignant mesothelioma does not show a distinct morphologic pattern and is typically composed of short storiform arranged fascicles akin to malignant fibrous histiocytoma or haphazardly arranged (so-called "patternless pattern" of) spindle cells as seen in solitary fibrous tumor (Figs. 10-22 and 10-23). The spindle cells may be arranged in long fascicles with a herringbone pattern imparting a fibrosarcomatous appearance. The cell nuclei are fusiform or plump and the cytoplasm eosinophilic. There may be some tumor giant cells. Variable amounts of necrosis and variable numbers of mitoses are seen. The stroma may be collagenous or myxoid. Inflammatory infiltrates are usually inconspicuous. Immunohistochemistry is generally less useful in the sarcomatoid as compared to the epithelioid form of diffuse malignant mesothelioma.[16–19] In some sarcomatoid diffuse malignant mesotheliomas, the tumor cells appear more plump and eosinophilic, imparting a leiomyosarcomatous appearance. Immunopositivity for smooth muscle actin and desmin occurs in about 9% of sarcomatoid diffuse malignant mesotheliomas.[17]

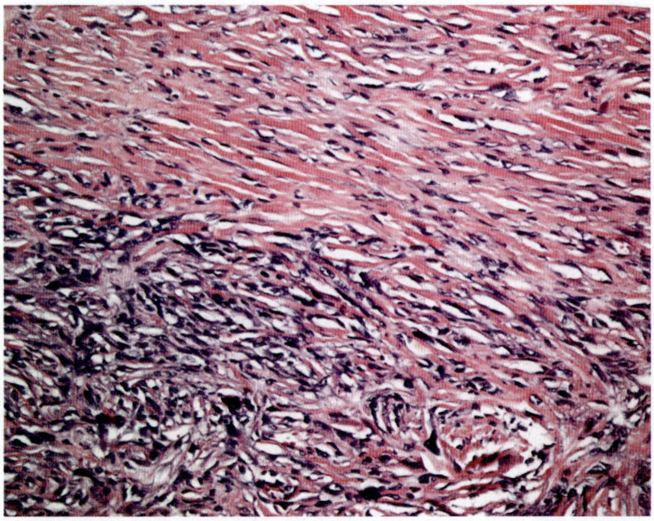

FIGURE 10-22: Diffuse malignant mesothelioma, sarcomatoid subtype, medium power.

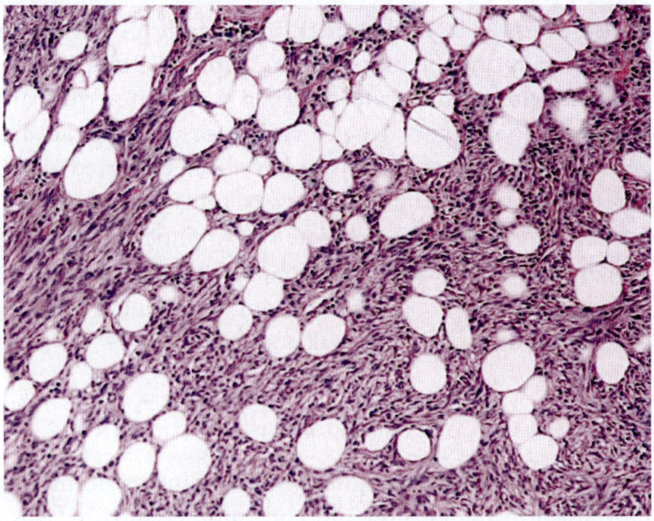

FIGURE 10-23: Diffuse malignant mesothelioma, sarcomatoid subtype, with tumor cells invading adipose tissue in a sieve-like (cribriform) pattern.

In a very small number of sarcomatoid diffuse malignant mesotheliomas, there is so-called heterologous differentiation into osteocartilaginous, rhabdomyosarcomatous, or liposarcomatous areas[18–20] (Figs. 10-14 to 10-27). These areas are frequently immunohistochemically inert.

The differential diagnosis includes organizing pleuritis, sarcomatoid carcinoma, metastatic sarcoma, metastatic melanoma, and solitary fibrous tumor. The clinical history (of known tumor elsewhere in the body) and anatomic distribution of the tumor are important considerations (localized versus diffuse). Immunohistochemistry is of limited use although broad-spectrum cytokeratin is useful to facilitate the identification of frank invasion (which excludes organizing pleuritis). Cytokeratin also excludes metastatic melanoma, most sarcomas, and solitary fibrous tumors (which are characteristically CD 34, BCL-2, and CD 99 positive). However, immunohistochemistry has very limited use in separating sarcomatoid carcinoma from sarcomatoid diffuse malignant mesothelioma or in separating synovial sarcoma from sarcomatoid diffuse malignant mesothelioma. Both nonmesothelial tumors have a tendency to be localized neoplasms. In addition, sarcomatoid carcinoma may show areas of

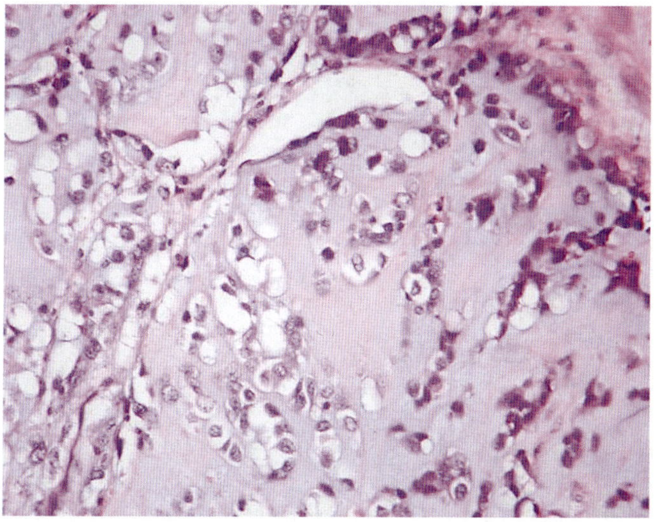

FIGURE 10-24: Diffuse malignant mesothelioma, sarcomatoid subtype, with heterologous (chondroid) differentiation.

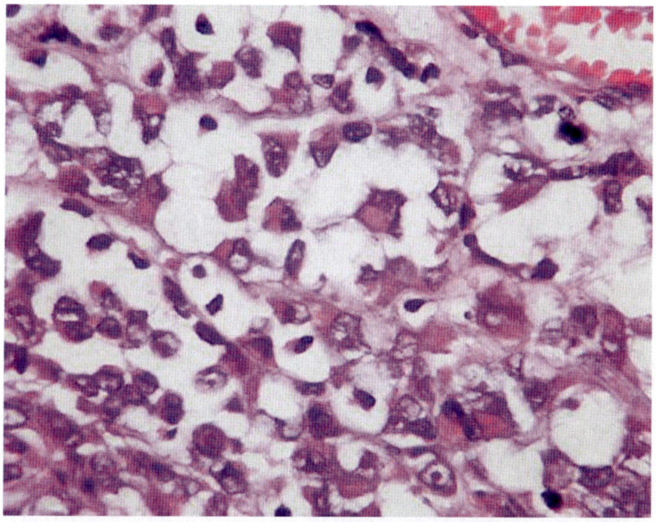

FIGURE 10-25: Diffuse malignant mesothelioma, sarcomatoid subtype, with heterologous (rhabdomyosarcomatous) differentiation.

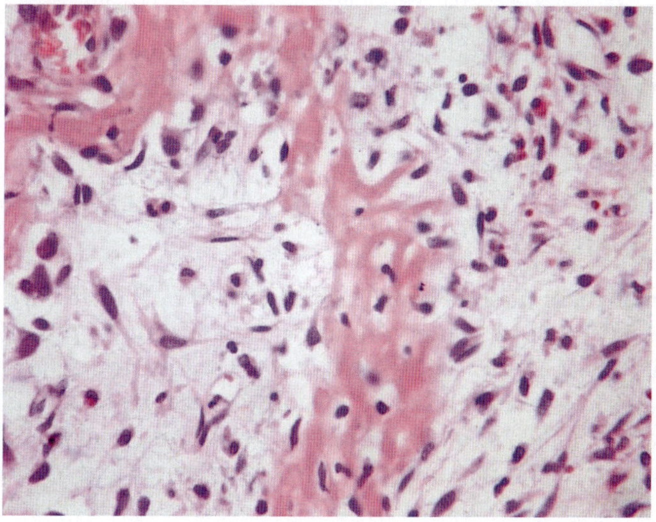

FIGURE 10-26: Diffuse malignant mesothelioma, sarcomatoid subtype, with heterologous (osteoid) differentiation.

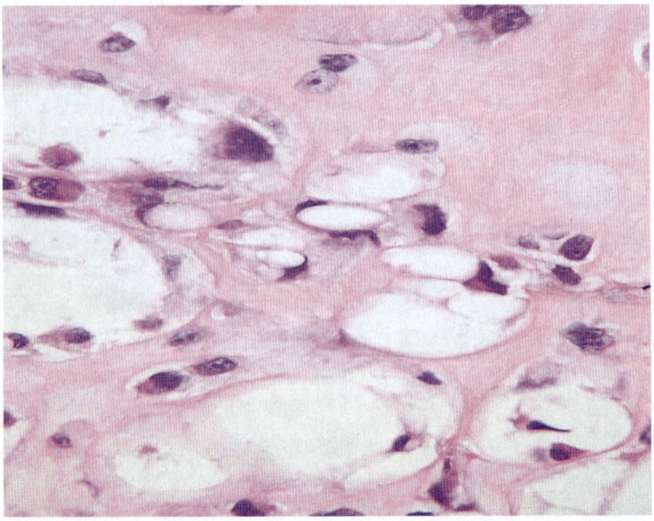

FIGURE 10-27: Diffuse malignant mesothelioma, sarcomatoid subtype, with lipoblast-like areas.

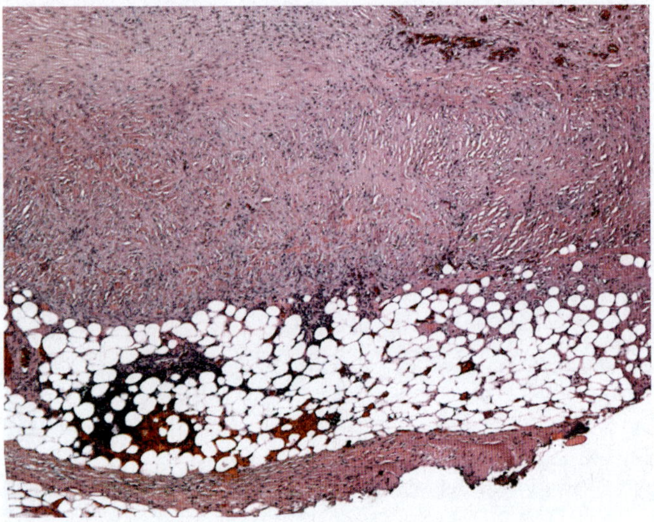

FIGURE 10-28: Diffuse malignant mesothelioma, desmoplastic. Low-power image.

epithelial (squamous or glandular) differentiation not seen in sarcomatoid diffuse malignant mesothelioma. Synovial sarcoma may be distinguished by cytogenetic analysis demonstrating the X:18 translocation. The translocation is observed in over 90% of cases and is not reported in diffuse malignant mesothelioma.

Desmoplastic Diffuse Malignant Mesothelioma

This form of sarcomatoid diffuse malignant mesothelioma is characterized by the presence of dense relatively bland collagenized tissue, which should occupy at least 50% of the tumor to conform to the WHO definition[1,21] (Figs. 10-28 and 10-29). It is notorious for its diagnostic confusion with organizing pleuritis. It is essentially never possible to make this diagnosis by needle biopsy. Although generally classified as a type of sarcomatoid diffuse malignant mesothelioma, a small number have been associated with the biphasic and epithelioid histologic patterns.

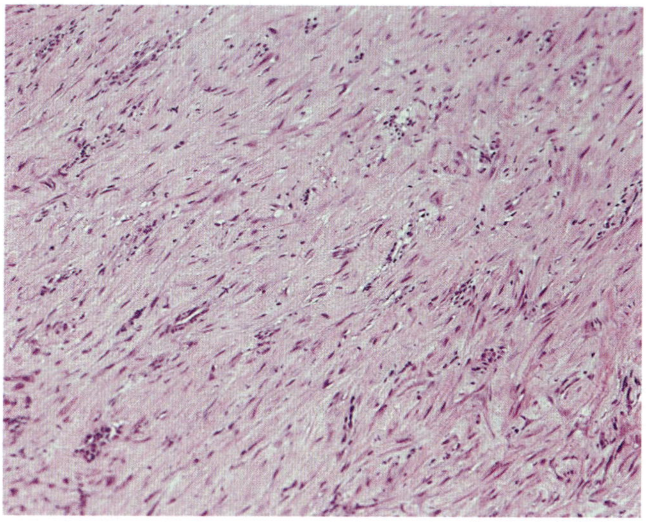

FIGURE 10-29: Diffuse malignant mesothelioma, desmoplastic. Paucicellular tumor, bland cytology, and abundant collagenous matrix mimic benign fibrous pleuritis.

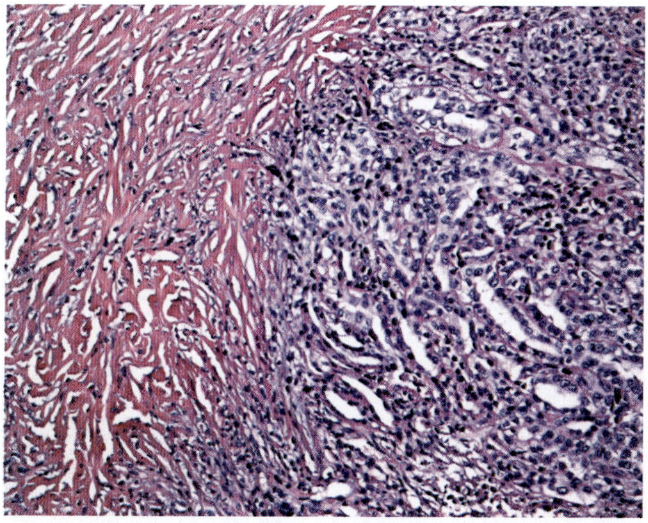

FIGURE 10-30: Diffuse malignant mesothelioma, biphasic subtype, with epithelioid component and desmoplastic sarcomatous component.

There are several criteria that are helpful in establishing the diagnosis of desmoplastic mesothelioma.[21] These are (1) foci of bland necrosis; (2) invasion of adipose tissue, skeletal muscle, or lung; (3) frankly sarcomatous areas; and (4) distant metastases. The latter can appear surprisingly bland. Cytokeratin staining may be helpful in identifying invasion.

Biphasic Diffuse Malignant Mesothelioma

Diffuse malignant mesotheliomas containing epithelioid and sarcomatoid components are designated biphasic by the WHO classification, providing each component comprises at least 10% of the tumor (Figs. 10-30 and 10-31). Any combination of patterns can occur. The proportion of cases classified as biphasic will go up with greater sampling of the tumor.

The differential diagnosis for biphasic diffuse malignant mesothelioma includes sarcomatoid carcinoma, carcinosarcoma (also malignant mixed mullerian tumors in the female peritoneum and mediastinum), biphasic synovial sarcoma, and malignant epithelioid vascular tumors, in particular epithelioid hemangioendothelioma (Figs. 10-32 and 10-33).

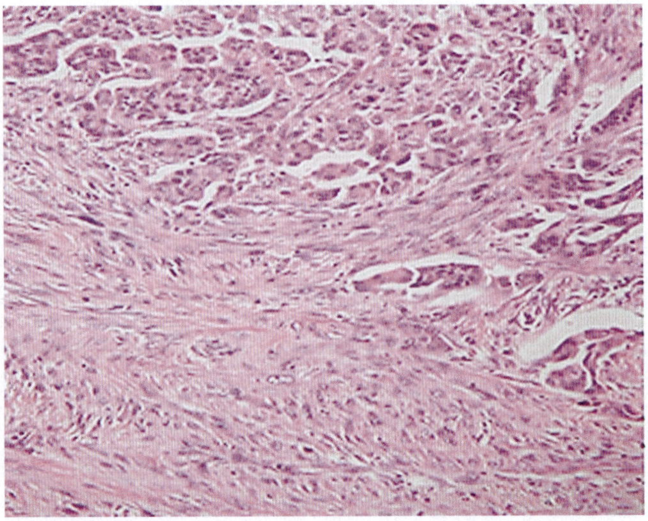

FIGURE 10-31: Diffuse malignant mesothelioma, biphasic subtype, with distinct epithelioid and sarcomatoid components.

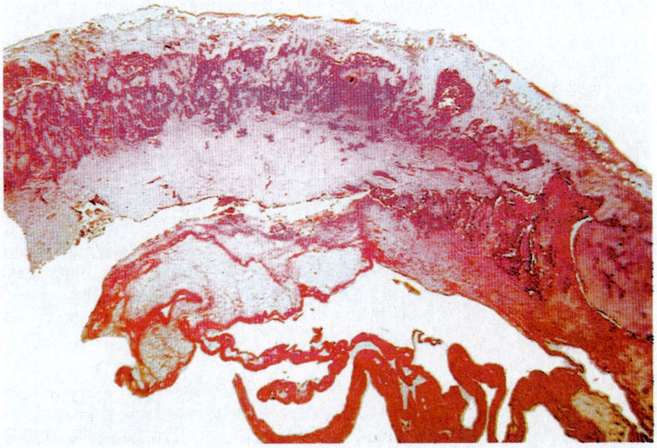

FIGURE 10-32: Epithelioid hemangioendothelioma with a diffuse growth pattern clinically mimicking pleural diffuse malignant mesothelioma.

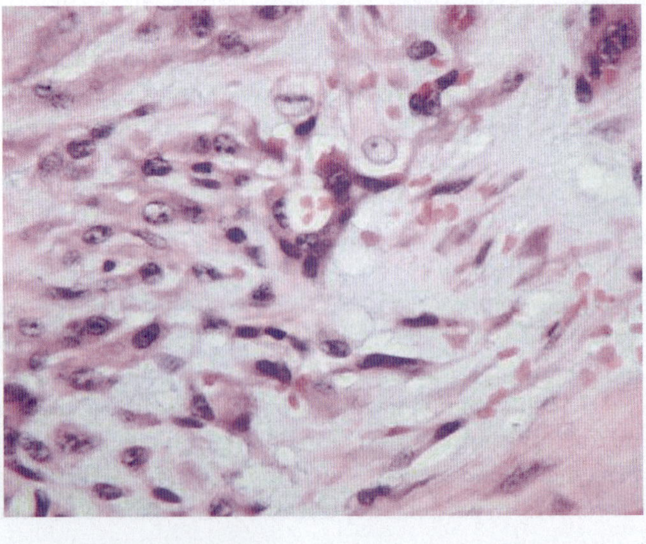

FIGURE 10-33: Epithelioid hemangioendothelioma. The tumor cells may be epithelioid or spindled and have small neovascular lumina present containing erythrocytes. There is often abundant myxohyaline stroma.

LOCALIZED MALIGNANT MESOTHELIOMA

Localized malignant mesotheliomas are extremely rare sharply circumscribed tumors of the serosal membranes with the microscopic appearance of diffuse malignant mesothelioma but lacking the diffuse growth pattern.[22] Fewer than 50 cases have been reported.[22–25] Localized malignant mesotheliomas have been described more frequently in the pleura than in the peritoneum or pericardium. The average age is approximately 60 years, and almost all patients are over 40 years of age. The sex ratio is 60:40 (male:female).[22] They are usually attached to the surface of the pleura, peritoneum, or pericardium in a sessile or pedunculated manner. They show a different biologic behavior to diffuse malignant mesothelioma, having a more favorable prognosis, and require different treatment.[22] At present an association with asbestos exposure is not proven. They may present as intrapulmonary masses, thus mimicking lung cancer.

WELL-DIFFERENTIATED PAPILLARY MESOTHELIOMA

It is important to separate well-differentiated papillary mesothelioma from conventional diffuse malignant mesothelioma because of its different demographics, different clinical behavior, and lack of association with asbestos exposure. It is very uncommon, reported most frequently in the peritoneum of women in the third and fourth decades of life, typically identified incidentally during surgical treatment for other conditions.[26–31] Rarely, it has been described in the pleura, pericardium, and tunica vaginalis.[32,33] A small number have been described in men. The majority behave in a benign or indolent fashion and are compatible with long survival. Some of the peritoneal cases have been managed with laparoscopic excision.[34] Very rare cases have been reported with a more aggressive course and progression to conventional diffuse malignant mesothelioma.[35] It is unclear whether all of these more aggressive tumors represent true well-differentiated papillary mesothelioma or if some represent undersampled diffuse malignant mesothelioma; however, cases of widely sampled and confidently diagnosed well-differentiated papillary mesothelioma, which over time have behaved more aggressively, have been encountered.

Grossly, well-differentiated papillary mesotheliomas are typically consist of small grey-white nodules, usually <2 cm in maximum dimension. The tumor is not characterized by the diffuse bulky spread of diffuse malignant mesothelioma. Histologically, it is characterized by a uniform well-defined complex papillary structure. Histologic criteria include (1) papillae lined by a single layer of bland cuboidal or columnar mesothelial cells with subnuclear vacuolation; (2) uniformity of tumor cells; (3) edematous or myxoid cores to the papillae, (iv) absence of nuclear features of malignancy and (v) absence of multilayering of cells in the papillary areas; (4) absent or minimal invasion; and (5) absent or rare mitoses (Figs. 10-34 to 10-36). There can be some irregularity of the tubulopapillary areas associated with fibrosis, and there can be solid areas, but these constitute a very small proportion of the tumor. The papillary lining cells stain appropriately with mesothelial immunohistochemical markers.

Well-differentiated papillary mesothelioma may be differentiated from diffuse malignant mesothelioma by the lack of a diffuse growth pattern, lack of cytologic atypia and cellular stratification, relative lack of invasion, and prominent uniform papillary architecture. However, differentiation may be impossible on small biopsies. The disease course is the ultimate discriminator, with few bona fide well-differentiated papillary mesotheliomas

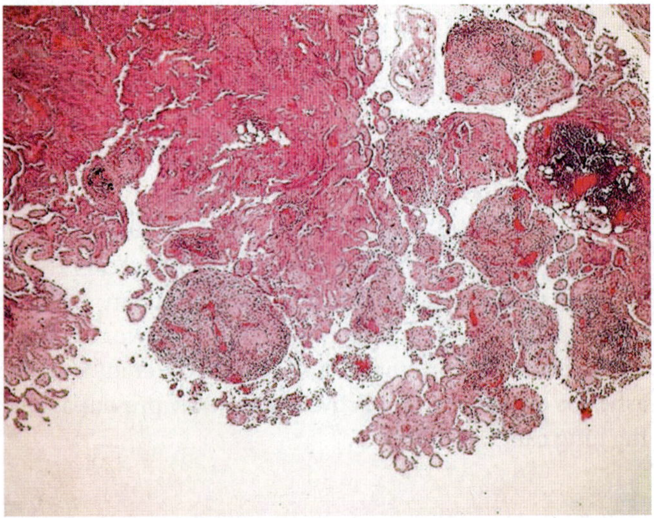

FIGURE 10-34: Well-differentiated papillary mesothelioma, with variable-sized papillae.

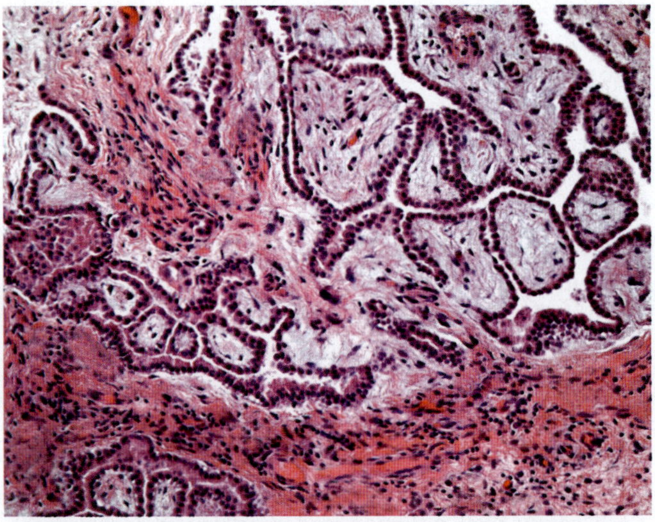

FIGURE 10-35: Well-differentiated papillary mesothelioma, medium power showing delicate papillary structures.

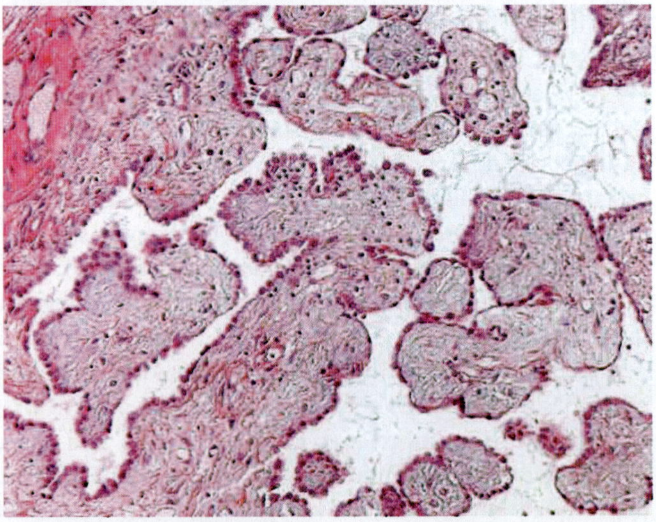

FIGURE 10-36: Well-differentiated papillary mesothelioma, higher power showing delicate papillary structures.

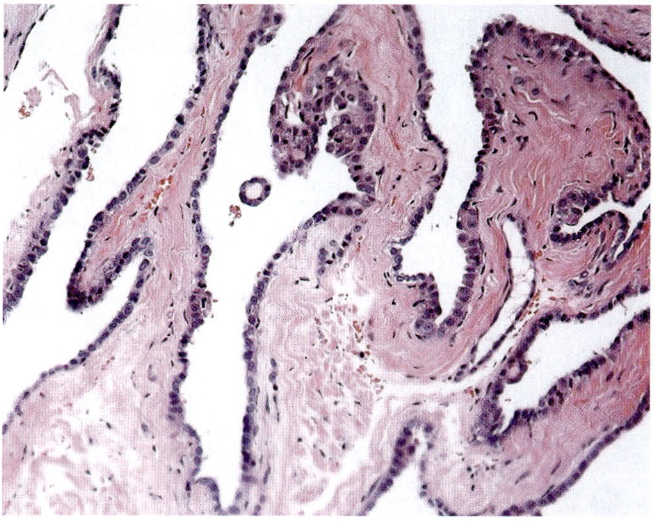

FIGURE 10-37: Reactive mesothelial hyperplasia with obvious papillary structures.

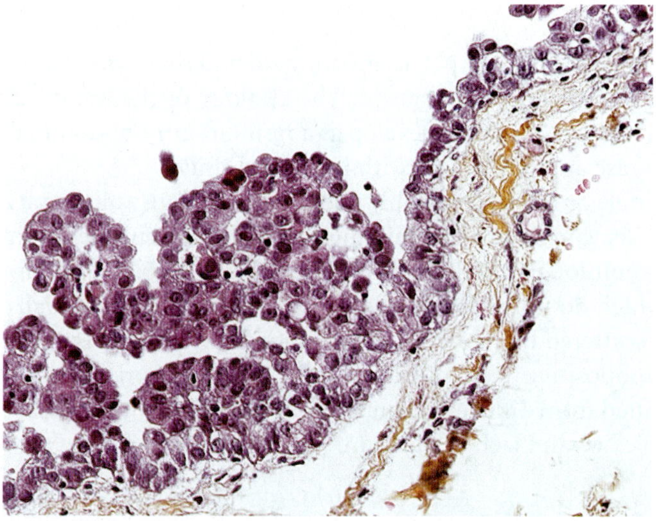

FIGURE 10-38: Diffuse malignant mesothelioma, with delicate solid epithelioid papillary structures.

progressing to a fatal outcome within a decade. Well-differentiated papillary mesothelioma may also be confused with reactive papillary mesothelial hyperplasia, a condition commonly seen in hernia sacs, and in the peritoneum associated with pelvic infection and endometriosis (Fig. 10-37). Some diffuse malignant mesotheliomas mimic well-differentiated papillary mesothelioma; however, the presence of solid epithelioid mesothelial papillary structures are an ominous predictor of malignancy (Fig. 10-38).

CYSTIC MESOTHELIOMA

Cystic mesothelioma and peritoneal inclusion cysts are alternative terms given to these lesions. They are comparatively rare and have been described most frequently in the peritoneum of reproductive age women and very rarely in the pleura. They are not associated with asbestos exposure. The majority are benign, but 30% to 50% recur following surgery and

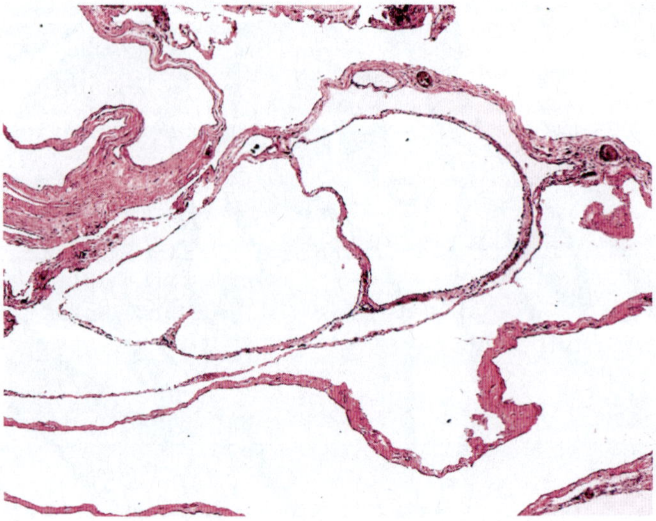

FIGURE 10-39: Cystic mesothelioma. (Reprinted from Shepherd NE, Warren BF, Williams GT, et al., eds. *Morson and Dawson's Gastrointestinal Pathology.* 5th ed. Oxford, UK: Wiley-Blackwell; 2013, with permission.)

rarely cause patient death.[36–42] Endometriosis and pelvic inflammatory disease frequently coexist with cystic mesotheliomas. They do not metastasize. The etiology of the lesions is unclear, although it has been postulated that that they develop as a result of intra-abdominal inflammation. The course of the disease appears to vary with hormonal shifts.

Grossly they are composed of single or multiple variably sized, smooth, thin-walled cysts that contain gelatinous fluid. The cysts vary from a few millimeters to several centimeters in size. Microscopically, the cysts are multilocular and lined by a single layer of bland cuboidal or flattened mesothelial cells, which do not show invasion (Fig. 10-39). The septal walls consist of fibrovascular tissue with scattered lymphocytes. In addition to mesothelial markers, there may be some focal immunopositivity with estrogen and progesterone receptors.[42] Cystic mesotheliomas are distinguished from diffuse malignant mesothelioma by their localized nature, lack of histologic complexity, and lack of invasion.

ADENOMATOID TUMOR

Adenomatoid tumors are benign lesions composed of mesothelial cells and are most frequently identified incidentally as minute nodules in the genital organs of men (epididymis and spermatic cord) and women (fallopian tube and uterus).[43] Rarely these tumors have been described in the omentum, mesentery, and pleura.[44–47] They usually measure <1 cm in diameter. Complete resection is curative.

Adenomatoid tumors are characterized by glandular spaces and papillae lined by large mesothelial cells and solid sheets with intracytoplasmic vacuoles (Fig. 10-40). The cells stain with the conventional immunohistochemical profile of mesothelial cells.[47] Cytologic atypia is absent. They may appear infiltrative microscopically, but they have an excellent prognosis.

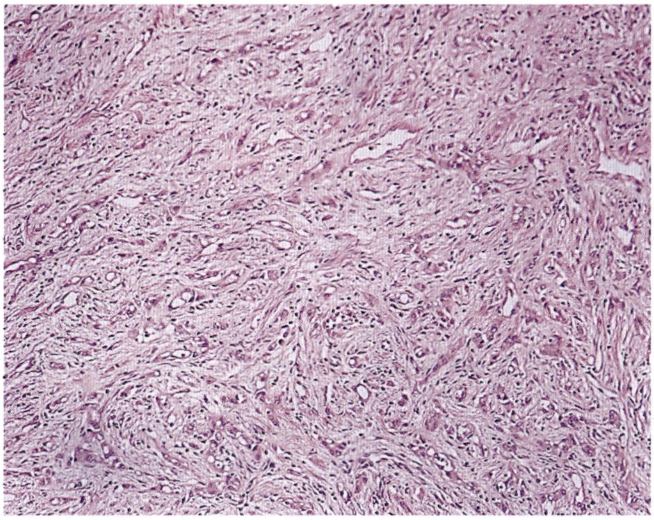

FIGURE 10-40: Adenomatoid tumor, with irregular infiltrative tubules mimicking epithelioid diffuse malignant mesothelioma. (Reprinted from Shepherd NE, Warren BF, Williams GT, et al., eds. *Morson and Dawson's Gastrointestinal Pathology*. 5th ed. Oxford, UK: Wiley-Blackwell, 2013, with permission.)

References

1. World Health Organization Classification of Tumours. In: Travis WD, Brambilla E, Muller-Hermelink HK, et al., eds. *Tumours of the Lung, Pleura, Thymus and Heart.* Lyon, France: IARC Press; 2004.
2. Churg A, Cagle PT, Roggli VL. Tumours of the serosal membranes. In: *Atlas of Tumour Pathology*, 4th series, fascicle 3. Washington, DC: Armed Forces Institute of Pathology; 2006:11–102.
3. Galateau-Salle F, ed. *Pathology of Malignant Mesothelioma. International Mesothelioma Panel.* London, UK: Springer; 2006.
4. Ordonez NG. Mesothelioma with clear cell features: an ultrastructural and immunohistochemical study of 20 cases. *Human Pathol* 2005;36:465–473.
5. Osborn M, Pelling N, Walker MM, et al. The value of "mesothelium-associated antibodies" in distinguishing between metastatic renal cell carcinomas and mesotheliomas. *Histopathology* 2002;41:301–307.
6. Mayall F, Gibbs AR. "Small cell" mesothelioma. *Histopathology* 1993;22:294–295.
7. Nascimento GA, Keeney GL, Fletcher CD. Deciduoid peritoneal mesothelioma: an unusual phenotype affecting young females. *Am J Surg Pathol* 1994;18:439.
8. Shanks JH, Harris M, Banerjee SS. Mesotheliomas with deciduoid morphology: a morphological spectrum and a variant not confined to young females. *Am J Surg Pathol* 2000;24:285.
9. Hammar SP, Bockus DE, Remington FL. Mucin positive epithelial mesotheliomas: a histochemical, immunohistochemical and ultra-structural comparison with mucin producing pulmonary adenocarcinoma. *Ultrastruct Pathol* 1996;20:293.
10. Cook DS, Attanoos RL, Jalloh SS. "Mucin positive" epithelial mesothelioma of the peritoneum: an unusual diagnostic pitfall. *Histopathology* 2000;17:33.
11. Joshi A, McAndrew N, Birdsall S, et al. Clear cell sarcoma mimicking malignant pleural mesothelioma *Histopathology* 2008;53:359–361.
12. Turc-Carel C, Aurias A, Mugneret F, et al. Chromosomes in Ewings' sarcoma an evaluation of 85 cases of remarkable consistency of t (11;22)(q24; q12). *Cancer Genet Cytogenet* 1988;32:229.
13. Gerald WL, Ladanyi M, de Alava E, et al. Desmoplastic small round-cell tumor: a recently recognized tumor type associated with a unique gene fusion. *Adv Anatomic Pathol* 1995;2:341–345.
14. Galateau-Salle F, Attanoos RL, Gibbs AR, et al. Lymphohistiocytoid variant of malignant mesothelioma of the pleura: a series of 22 cases. *Am J Surg Pathol* 2007;31:711–716.

15. Klebe S, Brownlee NA, Mahar A, et al. Sarcomatoid mesothelioma: a clinicopathologic correlation of 326 cases. *Mod Pathol* 2010:23;470–479.
16. Attanoos RL, Dojcinov S, Webb R, et al. Anti-mesothelial markers in sarcomatoid mesothelioma and other spindle cell neoplasms. *Histopathology* 2000;37:224–231.
17. Mayall FG, Goddard H, Gibbs AR. Intermediate filament expression in mesotheliomas: leiomyoid mesotheliomas are not uncommon. *Histopathology* 1992;2:453–457.
18. Attanoos RL, Webb R, Dojcinov SD, et al. Value of mesothelial and epithelial antibodies in distinguishing diffuse peritoneal mesothelioma in females from serous papillary carcinoma of the ovary and peritoneum. *Histopathology* 2002;40(3):237–244.
19. Klebe S, Mahar A, Henderson DW, et al. Malignant mesothelioma with heterologous elements: clinicopathological correlation of 27 cases and literature review. *Mod Pathol* 2008;21:1084–1094.
20. Lin BT, Colby T, Gown AM, et al. Malignant vascular tumours of the serous membranes mimicking mesothelioma. A report of 14 cases. *Am J Surg Pathol* 2002;20:1431.
21. Mangano WE, Cagle PT, Churg A, et al. The diagnosis of desmoplastic malignant mesothelioma and its distinction from fibrous pleurisy: a histologic and immunohistochemical analysis of 31 cases including p53 immunostaining. *Am J Pathol* 1998;110:191–199.
22. Allen TC, Cagle PT, Churg AM, et al. Localized malignant mesothelioma. *Am J Surg Pathol* 2005;29:866–873.
23. Crotty BT, Myers JL, Katzenstein AA, et al. Localized malignant mesothelioma. *Am J Surg Pathol* 1994;18:357–363.
24. Nakas A, Martin-Lucar AE, Edwards JG, et al. Localised malignant pleural mesothelioma: a separate clinical entity requiring aggressive local surgery. *Eur J Cardiothorac Surg* 2008;33:303–306.
25. Ascoli S, Dal Piaz G, Damiani S. Localised pleural malignant mesothelioma. Report of two cases simulating pulmonary carcinoma and review of the literature. *Virchows Archiv* 2004;445:206–209.
26. Daya D, McCaughey WT. Well differentiated papillary mesothelioma of the peritoneum. A Clinicopathologic study of 22 cases. *Cancer* 1990;65:292–296.
27. Goepel JR. Benign papillary mesothelioma of peritoneum: a histological, histochemical and ultrastructural study of six cases. *Histopathology* 1981;5:21–30.
28. Hoekman K, Tognon G, Risse EK, et al. Well-differentiated papillary mesothelioma of the peritoneum: a separate entity. *Eur J Cancer* 1996;32A:255–258.
29. Butnor K, Sporn TA, Hammar SP, et al. Well-differentiated papillary mesothelioma. *Am J Surg Pathol* 2001;25:1304–1309.
30. Galateau-Salle F, Vignaud JM, Burke L, et al. Well differentiated papillary mesotheliomas of the pleura: a series of 24 cases. *Am J Surg Pathol* 2004;28:534–540.
31. Kao S, Mahon K, Lin B, et al. Pleural well-differentiated papillary mesothelioma: a case report. *J Thorac Oncol* 2009;4:920–922.
32. Barbera V, Rubino M. Papillary mesothelioma of the tunica vaginalis. *Cancer* 1957;10:182–189.
33. Sane AC, Roggli VL. Curative resection of a well-differentiated papillary mesothelioma of the pericardium. *Arch Pathol Lab Med* 1995;119:266–267.
34. Nezhat FR, DeNoble SM, Brown DN, et al. Laparoscopic management of peritoneal mesothelioma associated with pelvic endometriosis. *J Minim Invasive Gynecol* 2010;17:646–650.
35. Foyle A, Al-Jabi M, McCaughey WT. Papillary peritoneal tumors in women. *Am J Surg Pathol* 1981;5:241–249.
36. Brimo F, Illei PB, Epstein JI. Mesothelioma of the tunica vaginalis: a series of eight cases with uncertain malignant potential. *Mod Pathol* 2010;23:1165–1172.
37. Weiss SW, Tavassolli FA. Multicystic mesothelioma: an analysis of pathological findings and biological behaviour in 37 cases. *Am J Surg Pathol* 1988;12:737–746.
38. Katsube Y, Mukai K, Silverberg SG. Cystic mesothelioma of the peritoneum: a report of five cases and review of literature. *Cancer* 1982;15:1615–1622.
39. Ross MJ, Welch WR, Scully RE. Multilocular peritoneal inclusion cysts (so-called cystic mesothelioma). *Cancer* 1989;64:1336–1346.

40. Ball NJ, Urbanski SJ, Green FH, et al. Pleural multicystic mesothelial proliferation. The so-called multicystic mesothelioma. *Am J Surg Pathol* 1990;14:375–378.
41. Vallerie AM, Lerner JP, Wright JD, et al. Peritoneal inclusion cysts: a review. *Obstet Gynecol Surv* 2009;64:321–334.
42. Sawn RN, Malpica A, Deaveres MT, et al. Benign cystic mesothelioma of the peritoneum: a clinicopathologic study of 17 cases and immunohistochemical analysis of estrogen and progesterone receptor status. *Hum Pathol* 2003;34:369–374.
43. Taxy JB, Battifora H, Oyasu R. Adenomatoid tumours: a light microscopic, histochemical and ultrastructural study. *Cancer* 1974;33:306–316.
44. Craig JR, Hart WR. Extragenital adenomatoid tumour. *Cancer* 1979;64:1336–1346.
45. Young RH, Silva EG, Scully RE. Ovarian and juxtaovarian adenomatoid tumours: a report of six cases. *Int J Gynecol Pathol* 1991;10:364–371.
46. Kaplan MA, Tazelaar HD, Hayashi T, et al. Adenomatoid tumours of the pleura. *Am J Surg Pathol* 1996;20:1219–1223.
47. Minato H, Nojima T, Kurose N, et al. Adenomatoid tumor of the pleura. *Pathol Int* 2009;59: 567–571.

Mucin Histochemistry and Electron Microscopy

11

Richard L. Attanoos

The morphologic diversity of diffuse malignant mesothelioma necessitates that the routine hematoxylin–eosin stains used for light microscopic diagnosis be complemented by ancillary studies such as mucin histochemistry, electron microscopy, and immunohistochemistry. The three ancillary diagnostic modalities may be summarized as most simple (histochemistry), most expensive (electron microscopy), and most widely applicable (immunohistochemistry). This chapter discusses the first—specifically, the role and limitations of mucin and ultrastructural studies in the diagnosis of diffuse malignant mesothelioma.

MUCIN HISTOCHEMISTRY

Mucin histochemistry is a simple, inexpensive method to use to aid in distinguishing diffuse malignant mesothelioma from adenocarcinoma. Its simplicity should not allow it to be overlooked in the rush to obtain immunostains. Diffuse malignant mesotheliomas contain glycogen and may produce hyaluronic acid, a nonsulfated anionic glycosaminoglycan produced by cell surface and internal membranes. Hyaluronic acid is produced by a variety of cells of epithelial and connective tissue histogenesis. It is produced by both normal and neoplastic mesothelial cells as well as a variety of nonmesothelial cells and tumor counterparts. Alcian blue, pH 2.5, and colloidal iron label hyaluronic acid on the cell surface or glandular space or as intracellular vacuoles (Fig. 11-1). This reaction may be abolished by pretreatment with hyaluronidase. It is customary to stain two slides, with and without hyaluronidase pretreatment such that comparisons may be made. Alcianophilic reactions stain blue, and this is markedly diminished or abolished after hyaluronidase treatment. Stromal hyaluronate serves as an internal control although it has no diagnostic application. Hyaluronic acid is water soluble, and prolonged fixation results in hyaluronate leaching in aqueous solutions yielding false-negative results. This effect may be prevented by using alcohol fixative. Nonetheless, equivocal results may occur, necessitating further ancillary, usually immunohistochemical, testing.

Adenocarcinomas may produce neutral mucin (Fig. 11-2). Periodic acid–Schiff (PAS) labels glycogen, basement membrane, lysosomes, leukocyte granules, and, importantly, neutral mucin. Diastase pretreatment removes glycogen, and the presence of diastase pretreated PAS droplets in tumor cells strongly favors neutral mucin deposition and adenocarcinoma. Because a significant number of adenocarcinomas do not produce neutral mucin and because there are technical problems with the reliability of labeling hyaluronic acid, the sensitivity of these techniques is relatively low—73% for diastase pretreated PAS and 41% for hyaluronidase pretreated Alcian blue pH 2.5.[1,2]

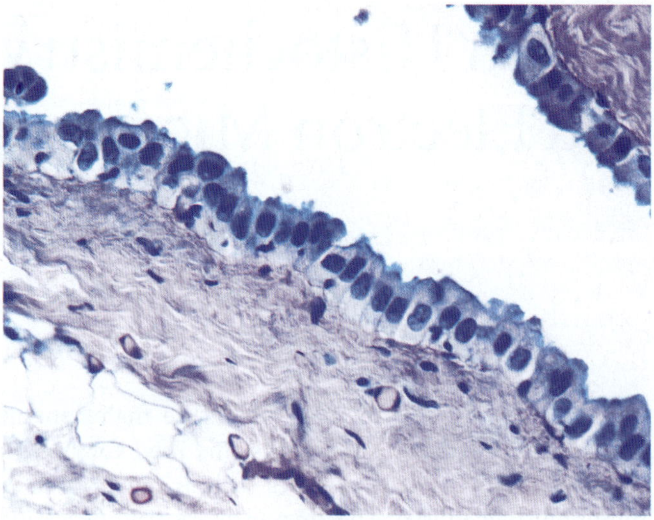

FIGURE 11-1: Alcian blue pH 2.5 stain in diffuse malignant mesothelioma with accentuated staining of hyaluronate on the cell surface.

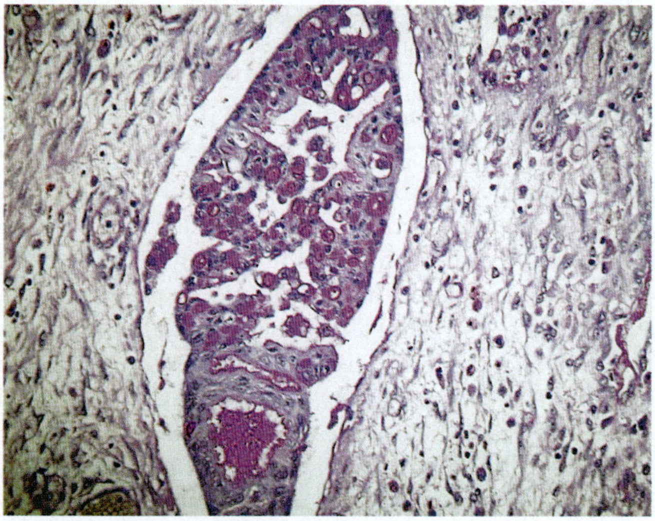

FIGURE 11-2: PAS stain with diastase pretreatment detecting neutral mucin in lung adenocarcinoma.

Additionally, there are recognized so-called "mucin-positive" epithelioid mesotheliomas in the pleura and peritoneum.[3,4] These are rare but otherwise typical diffuse malignant mesotheliomas, which are peculiarly defined by a number of unusual tinctorial staining patterns with mucin histochemistry. These tumors produce droplets of mucicarmine-positive, pretreated PAS-positive (Fig. 11-3), and hyaluronidase-resistant Alcian blue material. This mucin profile would ordinarily direct the pathologist to a diagnosis of adenocarcinoma. Moreover, immunophenotypically, these tumors may show a false-positive reaction with polyclonal carcinoembryonic antigen and CD 15 (Leu M1), further complicating the interpretation of the case.[5] However, positive mesothelial markers (such as calretinin, cytokeratin 5/6) are unchanged and positive, and the typical ultrastructural features of mesothelioma are present. Ultrastructurally, crystalline hyaluronate, visualized as scroll-like structures or "ferning" bodies (Fig. 11-4), has been postulated to be responsible for the unusual staining results.

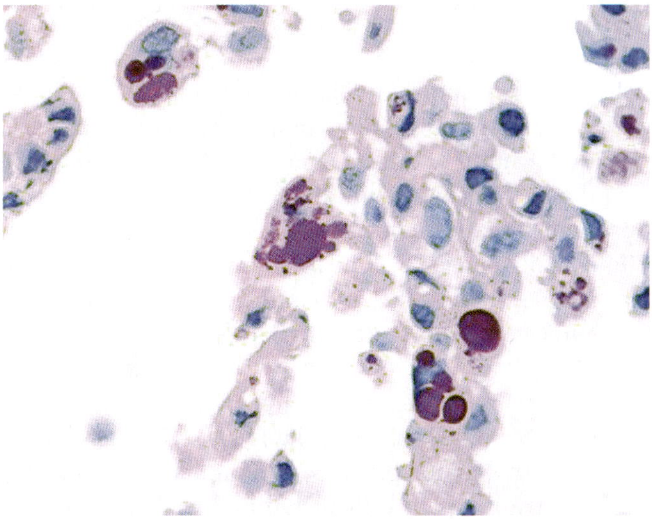

FIGURE 11-3: "Mucin"-positive epithelioid mesothelioma. Diastase pretreated PAS stain.

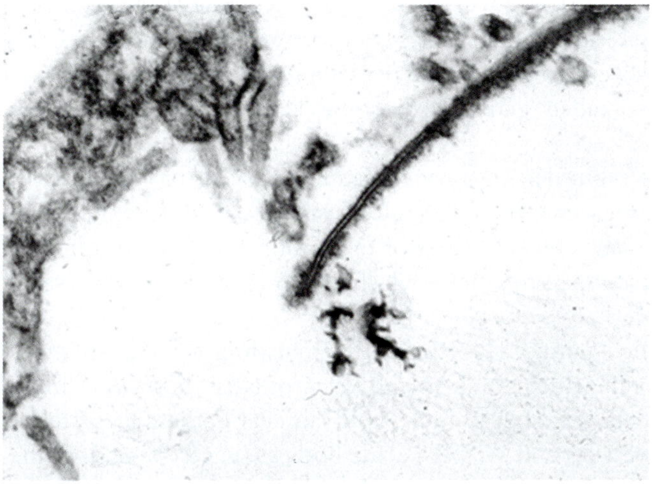

FIGURE 11-4: Diffuse malignant mesothelioma. Long microvilli and "ferning" bodies depicting crystalline hyaluronate in the "mucin"-positive epithelioid diffuse malignant mesothelioma. (Reprinted from Cook DS, Attanoos RL, Jalloh SS, et al., 'Mucin-positive' epithelial mesothelioma of the peritoneum: an unusual diagnostic pitfall. *Histopathology* 2000; 37:33–36, with permission.)

Mucin histochemistry also assists in distinguishing diffuse malignant mesothelioma from synovial sarcoma. Synovial sarcomas produce diastase-resistant PAS-positive (epithelial type) mucins, and these are also mucicarmine positive and hyaluronidase resistant. This contrasts with the acidic mucin production seen with diffuse malignant mesothelioma. Morphologic and immunophenotypic similarities exist between the two tumors; however, the relevance of mucin histochemistry is often understated in this setting with the emergence of molecular cytogenetics and the identification of the t(X;18) in over 90% synovial sarcomas. Because diffuse malignant mesothelioma is such an important tumor, with significant legal implications in the vast majority of cases, molecular cytogenetic testing should be performed in all suspected cases of synovial sarcoma. The role of mucin histochemistry is to facilitate the identification of those suspect cases for cytogenetic analysis.

ELECTRON MICROSCOPY

Electron microscopy has traditionally had an important role in the diagnosis of diffuse malignant mesothelioma and, via mineral analysis, continues to be significant to issues relating to tumor causation. The ultrastructural features of diffuse malignant mesothelioma have been extensively detailed, and without doubt the major application of this ancillary study is in the recognition of epithelioid diffuse malignant mesothelioma and its separation from adenocarcinoma and other epithelioid malignancies.[6–8] Electron microscopy has limited utility in distinguishing reactive from neoplastic mesothelial cells and from separating sarcomatoid mesothelioma from other spindle cell tumors such as sarcomas and sarcomatoid carcinomas.

The characteristic ultrastructural features of diffuse malignant mesothelioma are (1) microvilli, (2) tonofilaments, and (3) cell junction desmosomes (Table 11-1). Epithelioid diffuse malignant mesotheliomas are characterized by the presence of abundant long, slender, and often branching microvilli covering all surfaces of cells including inter- and intracellular lumina. These structures lack filamentous cores, core rootlets, and a surface glycocalyx. A microvillus size distribution ratio (length to width, >10:1) is considered predictive of diffuse malignant mesothelioma over adenocarcinoma. Tonofilaments are keratin intermediate filaments, which are often seen aggregated in fibrillary bundles converging at the cell membrane desmosomes or in the perinuclear regions. This pattern is rarely seen in adenocarcinoma. Cell junction desmosomes are present in diffuse malignant mesothelioma and other epithelial tumors. The presence of so-called "giant" desmosomes (>1 μm) is more predictive of diffuse malignant mesothelioma.

The ultrastructural presence of abundant intracytoplasmic glycogen may also be seen in cases of diffuse malignant mesothelioma. As the histologic subtype of diffuse malignant mesothelioma varies, so do the ultrastructural features of the tumor. Microvilli diminish in size and number as the tumor cell becomes sarcomatoid in shape, and the reverse occurs with increasing actin filament deposition.

The ultrastructural features, which point to a diagnosis other than diffuse malignant mesothelioma, are (1) cell surface microvilli, which are short and less profuse, with surface "fuzzy" glycocalyx formation and core rootlets, secretory granules, and lamellar bodies (suggestive of adenocarcinoma); (2) pinocytotic vesicles and Weibel-Palade bodies (suggestive of endothelial tumors such as epithelioid hemangioendothelioma and epithelioid angiosarcoma); and (3) melanosomes (seen in melanoma and some other pigmented tumors) (Table 11-2).

Table 11-1 Ultrastructural features characteristic of diffuse malignant mesothelioma

1. Microvilli	Abundant, long, slender Lack filamentous cores, core rootlets, and surface glycocalyx Microvillus length-to-width ratio >10:1
2. Tonofilaments	Converging at cell membrane desmosomes or in perinuclear regions
3. Cell junction desmosomes	Present; often "giant" desmosomes, >1 μm

Table 11-2	Ultrastructural features characteristic of tumors other than diffuse malignant mesothelioma
1. Cell surface microvilli	Short, less profuse, with "fuzzy" glycocalyx formation and core rootlets, secretory granules, and lamellar bodies
2. Pinocytotic vesicles	Suggest endothelial tumors and Weibel-Palade bodies
3. Melanosomes	Seen in melanoma and other pigmented tumors

Electron microscopy has some significant limitations. It is expensive and time consuming, and facilities are not widely available. Ultimately, this ancillary method for the diagnosis of diffuse malignant mesothelioma has been extensively replaced by more widely available and less expensive immunohistochemistry. Another significant limitation of electron microscopy that has led to its decreased use is that tissue, almost always fixed in formalin, requires subsequent reprocessing before electron microscopy can be performed. Finally, there are inevitable sampling problems with electron microscopy, which do not befall the other diagnostic modalities.

References

1. Roggli VL, Sanfilippo F, Shelburne JD. Mesothelioma. In: Roggli VL, Greenberg SD, Pratt PC, eds. *Pathology of Asbestos-Associated Diseases*. New York, NY: Little, Brown; 1992:109–153.
2. Cibas ES, Corson JM, Pinkus GS. The distinction of adenocarcinoma from malignant mesothelioma in cell blocks of effusions: the role of routine mucin histochemical assessment of carcinoembryonic antigen, keratin proteins, epithelial membrane antigen, and milk fat globule- derived antigen. *Hum Pathol* 1987;18:67–74.
3. Hammar SP, Bockus DE, Remington FL, et al. Mucin-positive epithelial mesotheliomas: a histochemical, immunohistochemical, and ultrastructural comparison with mucin-producing pulmonary adenocarcinomas. *Ultrastruct Pathol* 1996;20:293–325.
4. Cook DS, Attanoos RL, Jalloh SS, et al. 'Mucin-positive' epithelial mesothelioma of the peritoneum: an unusual diagnostic pitfall. *Histopathology* 2000;37:33–36.
5. Robb J. Mesothelioma versus adenocarcinoma: false-positive CEA and Leu-M1 staining due to hyaluronic acid. *Hum Pathol* 1989;20:400.
6. Warhol MJ, Hickey WF, Corson JM. Malignant mesothelioma: ultrastructural distinction from adenocarcinoma. *Am J Surg Pathol* 1982;6:307–314.
7. Oury TD, Hammar SP, Roggli VL. Ultrastructural features of diffuse malignant mesotheliomas. *Hum Pathol* 1998;29:1382–1392.
8. Hammar SP. Macroscopic, histologic, histochemical, immunohistochemical, and ultrastructural features of mesothelioma. *Ultrastruct Pathol* 2006;30:3–17.

Immunohistochemistry

12

Richard L. Attanoos

Immunohistochemistry plays a central role in the diagnosis of diffuse malignant mesothelioma. There is marked morphologic diversity in the tumor phenotype and mimicry of a number of histogenetically distinct tumors and also benign mesothelial proliferations. Over the past decade, in particular, there has been a vast expansion in the literature of comparative immunohistochemical studies involving diffuse malignant mesothelioma. It is questionable whether there is any other area of anatomic pathology in which immunohistochemistry has a higher profile. From the patient's and family's perspective, immunohistochemistry facilitates obtaining the correct diagnosis. This is important for both prognostic and legal reasons. From the pathologist's perspective, immunohistochemistry is important in facilitating the diagnosis, as the diagnosis of diffuse malignant mesothelioma is recognized to be difficult, especially in smaller and smaller tissue samples that are more routinely being obtained.

The plasticity of mesothelium has precluded the finding of a suitable single mesothelial epitope. As a consequence, efforts to produce a specific and sensitive mesothelial marker for use in formalin-fixed paraffin-embedded tissue have been unsuccessful; currently there exists no single antibody that is 100% specific and 100% sensitive for diffuse malignant mesothelioma.

As a general principle, it is important to apply a panel of antibodies that encompass expression across the range of differential diagnoses. The choice of antibodies to be incorporated into a panel is determined by the laboratory's and pathologist's experience and choice, the specific clinical diagnostic dilemma, the morphologic phenotype, and the anatomic site. In most cases, diffuse malignant mesothelioma diagnosis is considered in the pleural setting, but individual problems exist in the peritoneum, particularly in women.

There exist three main areas in which immunohistochemistry has a role in the diagnosis of malignant mesothelioma: (1) distinguishing malignant epithelioid neoplasms in the serosa; (2) distinguishing malignant sarcomatoid (spindle cell) neoplasms in the serosa; and (3) distinguishing reactive and neoplastic mesothelial proliferations, both epithelioid and spindle cell type.

ROLE OF IMMUNOHISTOCHEMISTRY IN DISTINGUISHING MALIGNANT EPITHELIOID NEOPLASMS

In serosal biopsy interpretation the most commonly encountered problem is distinguishing diffuse malignant mesothelioma of epithelioid subtype from metastatic adenocarcinoma. The tumor morphology is typically one or more of acinar, tubulopapillary, micropapillary, myxoid rich, or solid in type. A large number of immunomarkers have been proposed as having adjunct roles in the diagnosis of malignant mesothelioma in this setting.

The International Mesothelioma Panel proposes that two positive mesothelioma markers and two positive carcinoma markers together with a pancytokeratin are sufficient to allow for the distinction of diffuse malignant mesothelioma from metastatic carcinoma in the majority of cases.[1] Interlaboratory variations exist, and for various reasons, certain antibodies may be preferred; however, a proposed extended antibody panel should include four first-line positive mesothelial markers, calretinin, cytokeratin 5/6, WT1, and podoplanin (D2-40), together with six positive epithelial/carcinoma markers, carcinoembryonic antigen (CEA), Le M1 (CD15), Ber EP4, MOC-31, BG8, and thyroid transcription factor 1 (TTF-1). The strength and limitations of each marker are discussed below.

For certain malignant epithelioid proliferations in the pleura, the differential diagnosis lies between diffuse malignant mesothelioma of epithelioid subtype and a carcinoma exhibiting squamous cell or neuroendocrine differentiation. In the distinction of diffuse malignant mesothelioma and squamous carcinoma, the two preferred positive mesothelial markers are WT1 and calretinin, and the two preferred epithelial/carcinoma markers are p63 (or p40) and Ber EP4. For small cell diffuse malignant mesothelioma, the two preferred mesothelioma markers are calretinin and thrombomodulin, and the three preferred epithelial/carcinoma markers are CD56, CEA, and TTF-1. Occasional giant desmosomes are seen in rare epithelioid diffuse malignant mesotheliomas (often postirradiation cases), but bona fide keratinization is exceptional. Similarly, neuroendocrine differentiation in diffuse malignant mesothelioma is exceptional, and its presence should alert the pathologist to an alternate diagnosis.

DIFFUSE MALIGNANT MESOTHELIOMA, EPITHELIOID SUBTYPE: MORPHOLOGIC PATTERNS AND DIFFERENTIAL DIAGNOSES

For certain morphologic subtypes of diffuse malignant mesothelioma, other diagnostic considerations exist that prompt more extensive immunohistochemistry (Table 12-1). Due to the morphologic diversity of diffuse malignant mesothelioma of epithelioid subtype, certain cytoarchitectural patterns merit consideration of different differential diagnoses. For example, clear cell variant diffuse malignant mesothelioma mimics metastatic renal cell carcinoma (RCC) and clear cell carcinoma of the lung. Pleomorphic variant diffuse malignant mesothelioma mimics metastatic pleomorphic carcinoma of the lung, anaplastic carcinoma from other sites, malignant melanoma, and anaplastic large cell lymphoma. Lymphohistiocytoid variant diffuse malignant mesothelioma mimics metastatic lymphoepithelial carcinoma and non-Hodgkin lymphoma (Tables 12-2 to 12-5).

NOVEL AND ESTABLISHED MARKERS USED IN PANELS FOR MALIGNANT EPITHELIOID NEOPLASMS

Positive Epithelial/Carcinoma Markers

Carcinoembryonic Antigen

CEA is a glycoprotein involved in cell adhesion that is normally produced during fetal development. CEA positively labels between 70% and 100% of adenocarcinomas and seldom labels diffuse malignant mesothelioma cells. CEA is expressed in colorectal adenocarcinoma

Table 12-1 Morphologic variants of diffuse malignant mesothelioma

Malignant Mesothelioma	
Epithelioid	**Sarcomatoid**
Tubulopapillary	NOS, MFH
Microcystic/myxoid	Desmoplastic
Solid	Leiomyoid
Small cell	Heterologous
Lymphohistiocytoid	Lymphohistiocytoid
"Mucin" positive	
Clear cell	
Deciduoid	
Pleomorphic	
Transitional	

NOS, not otherwise specified; MFH, malignant fibrous histiocytoma-like.

Table 12-2 Distinguishing small cell diffuse malignant mesothelioma from its mimics

Small Cell Mesothelioma

Tumor	CK	CD45	Calretinin	Thr	CD56/CHR	Desmin
Mesothelioma	+	−	+	+	−	−/+
Small cell ca	+	−	−	−	+	−
NHL	−	+	−	−	CD56	−
DSRCT	−/+	−	−	+	NSE	+ (WT1)

CK, broad-spectrum cytokeratin; CD45, leukocyte common antigen; Thr, thrombomodulin; NHL, non-Hodgkin lymphoma; DSRCT, desmoplastic small round cell tumor; CD56, NCAM; NSE, neuron-specific enolase; CHR, chromogranin A; WT1, Wilms tumor susceptibility gene product 1.

Table 12-3 Distinguishing lymphohistiocytoid diffuse malignant mesothelioma and its mimics

Lymphohistiocytoid Mesothelioma

Tumor	CK	MESO	CD45	CD20	CD30	PLAP	Tdt
Mesothelioma	+	+	−	−	+/−	−	−
Thymoma	+	+	−	+	−	−	+(L)
Lymphoma	−	−	+	+	+	−	+
LE-like CA	+	−	−	−	−EBV	−	−
Dysgerminoma	−/+	−	−	−	+	+	−

CK, broad-spectrum cytokeratin; Thr, thrombomodulin; CD45, leukocyte common antigen; CD20, B lineage marker, also stains asteroid cells in thymoma; CD30, Ki 1 antigen, activation marker, most often positive in anaplastic large cell lymphoma and classical Hodgkin lymphoma; PLAP, placental alkaline phosphatase; Tdt, terminal deoxynucleotidyl transferase, positive in lymphoblastic lymphoma/leukemia, also pre–T lymphocytes in thymic epithelial tumors; LE, lymphoepithelioma; CA, carcinoma; EBV, Ebstein-Barr virus; MESO, cytokeratin 5/6, thrombomodulin, calretinin.

Table 12-4 Distinguishing pleomorphic carcinoma and its mimics

Pleomorphic Mesothelioma					
Tumor	**CK**	**CD45**	**Calretinin**	**HMB-45/S100**	**Epithelial**
Mesothelioma	+	–	+/–	+/–	–/+
Anaplastic carcinoma	+	–	–/+	–	+/–
Anaplastic lymphoma	–	+	–	–	–
Melanoma	–	–	–	+	–

Epithelial markers: CEA, MOC-31, CD15, BG 8, Ber EP4. Note that EMA may be expressed in all of the above tumors and is of no diagnostic value in these cases and should not be used.

Table 12-5 Distinguishing clear cell diffuse malignant mesothelioma and its mimics

Clear Cell Mesothelioma					
Tumor	**CK**	**"MESO"**	**CD45**	**HIM-45**	**PLAP**
Mesothelioma	+	+	–	–	–
Clear cell carcinoma	+	+	–	+	–
Lymphoma	–	–	+	–	+
Clear cell sarcoma	–	–	–	+	–
Dysgerminoma	–/+	–	–	–	+
PECOMA	–	–	–	+	–

"MESO": cytokeratin 5/6, thrombomodulin, (calretinin) markers (a small proportion of RCCs express all mesothelial markers, also RCC marker reported in <10% mesotheliomas.)
Lymphoma: Clear cell differentiation reported in various lymphomas notably primary sclerosing mediastinal lymphoma (formerly clear cell lymphoma), peripheral T-cell lymphoma, plasma cell tumors, marginal zone lymphoma (monocytoid appearance)
Clear cell sarcoma (melanoma of soft parts) associated with EWSR-1 ATF-1 gene
PECOMA: perivascular endothelioid cell tumor also labels with melan-A (MITF), actin, myosin, and calponin.

(Fig. 12-1), gastric adenocarcinoma, pancreatic adenocarcinoma, lung adenocarcinoma, breast carcinoma, and medullary thyroid carcinoma. Polyclonal antibodies to CEA are recognized to produce false-positive staining in diffuse malignant mesothelioma due to reactivity with nonspecific cross-reactive antigen. Monoclonal CEA has higher specificity and less sensitivity for adenocarcinoma than does polyclonal CEA. In one study, polyclonal CEA was found to have 83% sensitivity and 95% specificity for adenocarcinoma.[2] Polyclonal CEA is generally the preferred marker on account of its higher sensitivity. A systematic review of 51 studies (consisting 1,524 pulmonary adenocarcinomas and 1,818 diffuse malignant mesotheliomas of epithelioid subtype) reported 83% sensitivity and 95% specificity for CEA. In 24 studies, monoclonal CEA was used (incorporating 949 pulmonary adenocarcinomas and 1,007 diffuse malignant mesotheliomas, epithelioid subtype) with an estimated 81% sensitivity and 97% specificity[3–6] (Table 12-6).

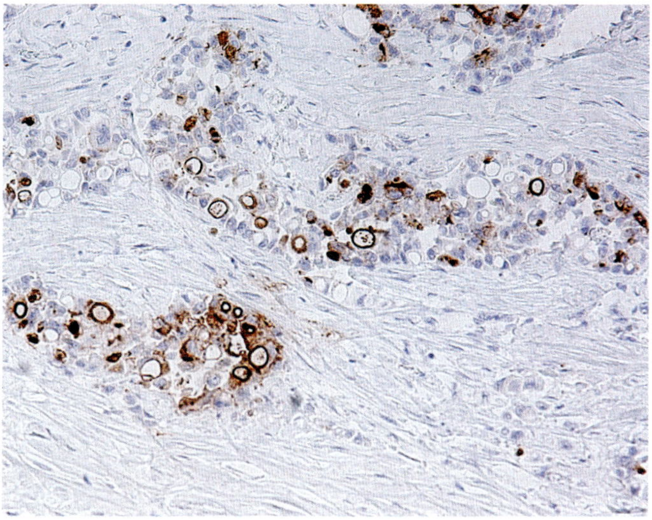

FIGURE 12-1: CEA expression in adenocarcinoma.

Leu M1 (CD15)

Leu M1 (CD15) is a sugar moiety component of an adhesion molecule expressed on glycoproteins, glycolipids, and proteoglycans. In immunohistochemistry, it has been most commonly used to identify myelomonocytic lineage cells and Reed-Sternberg cells in Hodgkin lymphoma. It is also recognized that Leu M1 labels over 60% of adenocarcinomas with both membranous and cytoplasmic expressions. Leu M1 was identified to have a 72% sensitivity and 93% specificity for pulmonary adenocarcinoma in a meta-analysis study by King.[2]

Ber EP4

Ber EP4 was derived from the breast cancer cell line MCF-7 and labels the majority of adenocarcinomas. Ber EP4 has been reported to be expressed on various epithelial cells, except the superficial layers of squamous epithelium, hepatocytes, and parietal cells. It is not usually

Table 12-6 Laboratory comparisons of polyclonal and monoclonal CEA in adenocarcinoma and diffuse malignant mesothelioma

Author	Adenocarcinoma	Malignant Mesothelioma
Sheibani et al.[3]	38/50 (76%)^{P} 36/50 (72%)^{M}	0/28 (0%)^{P,M}
Otis et al.[4]	10/14 (71%)^{P} 9/14 (64%)^{M}	2/19 (11%)^{P} 6/19 (32%)^{M}
Dejmek and Hjerpe[5]	20/20 (100%)^{M} 15/20 (75%)^{M*} 16/20 (80%)^{M**} 16/20 (80%)^{M***}	13/61 (21%)^{P} 0/61 (0%)^{M*} 7/61 (11%)^{M**} 1/61 (2%)^{M***}
Bateman et al.[6]	10/14 (71%)^{P} 10/14 (71%)^{M}	2/17 (12%)^{P} 0/17 (0%)^{M}

P, polyclonal CEA; M, monoclonal CEA; M*, monoclonal antibody clone A5 B7; M**, monoclonal CEA clone CEJ 065; M***, monoclonal CEA clone SP651.

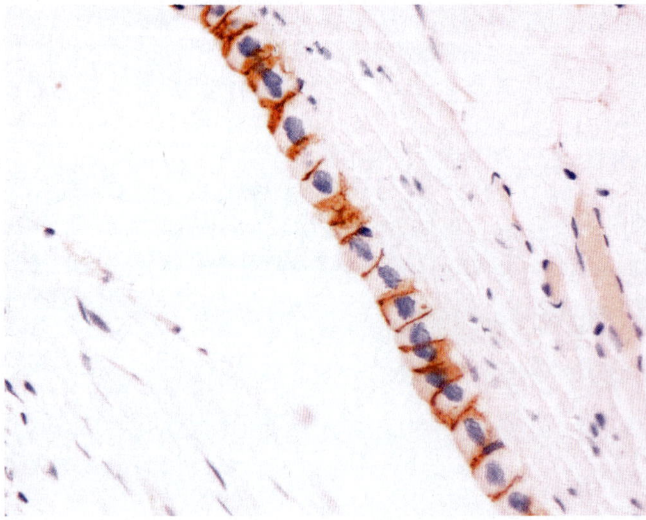

FIGURE 12-2: Lateral membrane expression of Ber EP4 in diffuse malignant mesothelioma. A potential pitfall.

expressed in diffuse malignant mesotheliomas; however, up to 20% of diffuse malignant mesotheliomas may show focal expression, usually membranous staining[7–10] (Fig. 12-2). In a systematic review of 17 studies (consisting of 702 pulmonary adenocarcinomas and 899 epithelioid diffuse malignant mesotheliomas), reported sensitivities and specificities of Ber EP4 for pulmonary adenocarcinoma were 80% and 90%, respectively.[2] Ber EP4 has a lower rate of positivity in nonpulmonary adenocarcinomas, expressed in 35% to 50% of RCCs (Table 12-7).

MOC-31

MOC-31 was raised against neuraminidase-treated cells from small cell carcinoma. It is expressed in a wide range of carcinomas. Its primary role is to distinguish adenocarcinomas (Fig. 12-3) from epithelioid diffuse malignant mesotheliomas, which are usually negative. The systematic review of seven studies consisting of 213 pulmonary adenocarcinoma and 276 epithelioid diffuse malignant mesotheliomas reported 93% sensitivity and 93% specificity for pulmonary adenocarcinoma.[2]

Thyroid Transcription Factor 1

TTF-1 is a 38-kDa nuclear transcription protein, which serves as a master regulator gene, which is required for thyroid-specific gene expression and development of surfactant apoproteins.

Table 12-7 Ber EP4 expression in adenocarcinoma and epithelioid diffuse malignant mesothelioma

Author	Adenocarcinoma	Diffuse Malignant Mesothelioma
Sheibani et al.[7]	72/83 (87%)	1/115 (0.9%)
Gaffey et al.[8]	103/120 (86%)	10/49 (20%)
Dejmek et al.[9]	28/43 (65%)	14/110 (13%)
Ordonez[10]	101/110 (92%)	18/70 (26%)

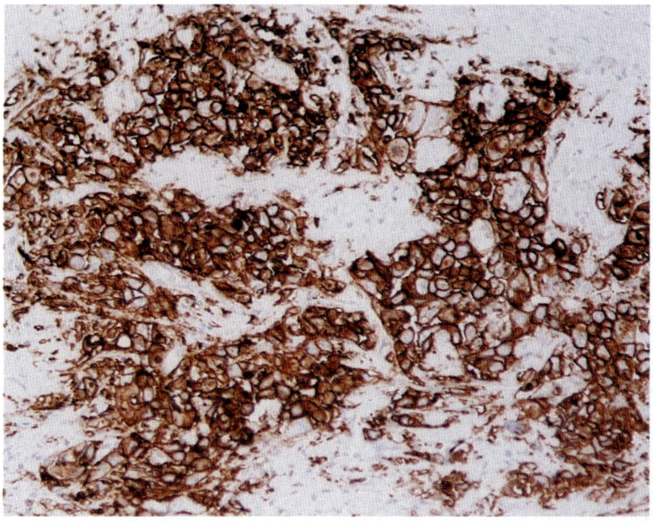

FIGURE 12-3: MOC-31 expression in adenocarcinoma, showing strong cytoplasmic elaboration.

TTF-1 is expressed in various normal tissues including follicular cells of the thyroid, parathyroid gland cells, parafollicular C cells, pituicytes, and type 2 pneumocytes. TTF-1 is commercially available as a monoclonal antibody 8G7G3/1 or with greater sensitivity and less specificity as SPT 24. Polyclonal antibodies to TTF-1 exist with lower sensitivity. TTF-1 has an important role as a positive marker of pulmonary adenocarcinoma and small cell carcinoma (where it is expressed in ~80% of cases). There is a higher reported rate of TTF-1 expression in primary pulmonary adenocarcinomas derived from the terminal respiratory unit, that is, acinar, lepidic, and papillary patterns of adenocarcinoma. TTF-1 expression is nuclear in distribution. Occasional cases report granular cytoplasmic expression that is regarded as nonspecific. Cytoplasmic TTF-1 expression is due to cross-reacting antigen and is usually granular in nature. In a systematic review of five studies (consisting of 366 pulmonary adenocarcinoma and 240 malignant mesotheliomas of epithelioid subtype), TTF-1 had a reported 72% sensitivity and 100% specificity for pulmonary adenocarcinoma.[2] In contrast, only 5% of squamous cell carcinomas of the lung are positive for TTF-1. TTF-1 is expressed in approximately 50% of large cell neuroendocrine carcinomas. To date, there is no reported expression of TTF-1 in diffuse malignant mesothelioma.

BG8

BG8 is a monoclonal antibody that recognizes the Lewis blood group antigen. In a meta-analysis of three studies consisting of 231 pulmonary adenocarcinomas and 197 epithelioid diffuse malignant mesotheliomas, BG8 clone had a reported 93% sensitivity and 93% specificity for pulmonary adenocarcinoma.[2]

Intermediate Filaments

The intermediate filaments represent a supergene family of proteins that measure between 7 and 22 nm in diameter and share common structural in sequence features.[11] There are six classified subtypes of intermediate filaments, and types 1 to 4 have been investigated with reference to the diagnosis of diffuse malignant mesothelioma (Table 12-8). In a meta-analysis by King of 88 comparative immunohistochemical studies, calretinin was observed to have 82% sensitivity and 85% specificity for epithelioid diffuse malignant mesothelioma.[2]

Table 12-8 Intermediate filament groups in mammalian systems

Type	Comments
1	Acidic cytokeratins (CK9-20)
2	Basic cytokeratins (CK1-8)
3	Desmin, glial fibrillary acidic protein, peripherin, vimentin
4	Alpha internexin, neurofilaments, synemin, syncoilin
5	Nuclear lamins
6	Nestin

Cytokeratins

Cytokeratins are intracytoplasmic skeletal proteins of epithelial tissue and are usually found in pairs comprising acidic type 1 and basic type 2 cytokeratin pairs. Almost all epithelial cells express cytokeratins and their expressions are frequently organ or tissue specific. Cytokeratin profiling by immunohistochemistry has been widely used for tumor diagnosis.

Normal and neoplastic mesothelial cells express low and high molecular weight cytokeratins. In diffuse malignant mesothelioma, epithelioid subtype, the cytokeratin filaments are in high density and arranged as concentric perinuclear bundles. These can be highlighted by the use of a broad-spectrum or pankeratin marker such as AE1/AE3.

Type 2 Intermediate Filament: Cytokeratin 5/6

Cytokeratin 5/6 is expressed in normal and neoplastic mesothelial cells and reported as a marker of diffuse malignant mesothelioma in 1989.[12] Immunoreactivity was identified in 12/13 (92%) of diffuse malignant mesotheliomas with no expression in any of the pulmonary adenocarcinomas tested. The original monoclonal antibody AE14 is applicable only in frozen section material and has limited use. In the mid-1990s, cytokeratin 5/6 antibody became commercially available for use in formalin-fixed paraffin-embedded material. Various studies have reported between 90% sensitivity and 85% specificity differentiating epithelioid diffuse malignant mesotheliomas from pulmonary adenocarcinomas[2,10,12–14] (Table 12-9).

Table 12-9 Expression of cytokeratin 5/6 in diffuse malignant mesothelioma

Author	Specificity (%)	Sensitivity (%)
Moll et al.[12]	92	100
Clover et al.[13]	85	100
Ordonez et al.[10]	85	100
Cury et al.[14]	86	92
King et al.[2]	85	83

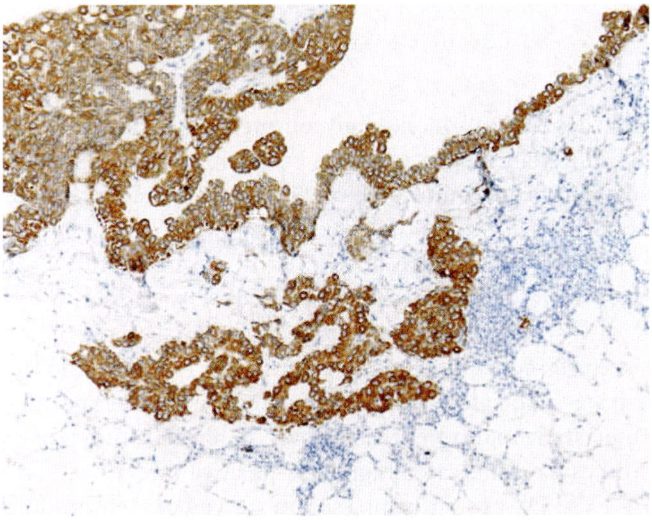

FIGURE 12-4: Cytokeratin 5/6 expression in epithelioid diffuse malignant mesothelioma, showing strong cytoplasmic expression.

In a meta-analysis study summarizing 88 published papers comparing immunohistochemical markers used in the diagnosis of epithelioid diffuse malignant mesothelioma, cytokeratin 5/6 sensitivity was 83% with 85% specificity.[2] Overall, cytokeratin 5/6 is recognized to be a first-line marker used in discriminating epithelioid diffuse malignant mesothelioma from pulmonary adenocarcinoma (Fig. 12-4). It is important to remember that because cytokeratin 5/6 is expressed in squamous-derived epithelium and derivative malignant counterpart carcinomas, cytokeratin 5/6 is expressed in squamous cell carcinoma and transitional cell carcinoma. As a consequence, cytokeratin 5/6 expression is almost constantly identified in these epithelia and tumors, and cannot be used to discriminate between epithelioid diffuse malignant mesothelioma and squamous cell carcinoma or transitional cell carcinoma.[15]

Type 3 Intermediate Filaments: Vimentin and Desmin

Vimentin filaments are present in most normal and neoplastic cells of mesenchymal origin including normal submesothelial cells but not resting surface mesothelium. In diffuse malignant mesothelioma vimentin can be identified in almost all cases. Because of its widespread distribution among tissues and tumors, vimentin has low specificity; and as a consequence, it is no longer used as a marker for diffuse malignant mesothelioma. A systematic meta-analysis of 17 studies, consisting of 773 epithelioid diffuse malignant mesotheliomas and 815 pulmonary adenocarcinomas, reported 62% sensitivity and 75% specificity of vimentin for diffuse malignant mesothelioma.[2] Vimentin antibodies may be used to test retained tissue antigenicity in cases in which there is suspected delay in fixation and other immunohistochemical tests are unusually negative. Positive vimentin expression demonstrates retained antigenicity.

Desmin is a marker of smooth and striated muscle; its primary role is in the separation of reactive from neoplastic mesothelial proliferations, discussed below.

Other type 3 intermediate filaments (glial fibrillary acidic protein) and type 4 intermediate filaments (neurofilaments) have been studied and found not to be expressed in diffuse malignant mesothelioma.[16]

Cell Surface Glycoproteins

Cadherins

Cadherins are transmembrane "calcium-dependent adhesion" glycoprotein. There are multiple classes of cadherin molecule, and the different members of the cadherin family are found in different tissues. For example, E-cadherins are found in epithelial tissue, N-cadherins are found in neuronal tissue, and P-cadherins are found in the placenta.

N-cadherin has been reported in pleural mesothelial cells and diffuse malignant mesothelioma. In a meta-analysis study by King, the reported expression of N-cadherin was associated with 78% sensitivity and 84% specificity in epithelioid diffuse malignant mesotheliomas.[2] In contrast, E-cadherin is expressed by lung epithelial cells and adenocarcinoma. In the same meta-analysis, E-cadherin was associated with 86% sensitivity and 82% specificity for pulmonary adenocarcinoma metastatic to the pleura. However, published studies have yielded conflicting results.[17] Some studies have indicated high false-positive rates of cadherins in both tumors. N-cadherin is a 135-kDa protein expressed in nerve cells, embryonic skeletal muscle, cardiac myocytes, and pleural mesothelial cells. Expression of N-cadherin was identified in all histologic subtypes of malignant mesothelioma but was most prominent in the epithelioid subtype. N-cadherin requires further evaluation, and other positive mesothelial markers have been more fully evaluated and shown to demonstrate higher specificity and sensitivity for diffuse malignant mesothelioma. As a consequence, the use of N-cadherin as a positive marker for diffuse malignant mesothelioma is not advocated at present.

Vascular Cell Adhesion Molecule-1

Vascular cell adhesion molecule-1 (VCAM-1) is a cytokine-inducible adhesion molecule, which recognizes ligands on leukocytes and has been reported in diffuse malignant mesothelioma cell lines in 14/16 (88%) diffuse malignant mesotheliomas (7 epithelioid, 8 biphasic, and 1 sarcomatoid subtype). Intercellular adhesions molecule-1 was diffusely expressed in all cases. VCAM-1 was expressed in 1/58 (1.7%) of various carcinomas.[18]

Thrombomodulin (CD141)

Thrombomodulin is a 75-kDa transmembrane glycoprotein, which functions as a cofactor in the thrombin-induced activation of protein C in the anticoagulant pathway. It is expressed in a limited array of human tissues including endothelial cells, platelets, syncytiotrophoblast, and mesothelial cells. Thrombomodulin was initially reported as a highly sensitive and specific marker in distinguishing pleural mesothelioma from pulmonary adenocarcinoma.[19] Subsequent investigators reported approximately 60% to 80% sensitivity and 33% to 94% specificity.[20–22] The meta-analysis review of 16 studies, consisting of 831 epithelioid diffuse malignant mesotheliomas and 964 pulmonary adenocarcinomas, reported 61% sensitivity and 80% specificity of thrombomodulin for diffuse malignant mesothelioma.[2] Published studies report no significant difference in thrombomodulin expression in either pleural or peritoneal cases although the marker has lower utility in the peritoneum due to its expression in over one-third of both serous papillary carcinomas of the ovary and peritoneum.[23] Thrombomodulin is expressed in both reactive and neoplastic mesothelial cells. As a consequence it plays no role in distinguishing benign and malignant mesothelial proliferations.

Thrombomodulin is best regarded as a second-line mesothelial marker due to its relatively low sensitivity for epithelioid diffuse malignant mesothelioma and very limited utility in sarcomatoid diffuse malignant mesothelioma. However, there is evidence that thrombomodulin may be preferentially expressed in small cell diffuse malignant mesothelioma.[24] Prominent membranous expression is common in diffuse malignant mesothelioma (Fig. 12-5). Interpretive problems exist with thrombomodulin as a result of its expression in endothelium. The surgical pathologist should be cautious about overinterpreting very focal linear and noncircumferential thrombomodulin staining, especially in proposed sarcomatoid diffuse malignant mesothelioma cases. The same interpretive problem is encountered with D2-40 (podoplanin). Because thrombomodulin and D2-40 are expressed in endothelium, staining within bona fide epithelioid vascular sarcomas may lead the unwary pathologist to misdiagnose diffuse malignant mesothelioma. In this setting, it is important to examine pancytokeratin staining, as most epithelioid vascular sarcomas are cytokeratin negative, and those that are positive show low-intensity focal expression, which contrasts with the high-intensity diffuse expression seen in bona fide epithelioid diffuse malignant mesothelioma. Thrombomodulin (together with cytokeratin 5/6) is typically expressed in squamous epithelial cells and its tumors, urothelial cells and its tumors, and in other tumors, which may mimic diffuse malignant mesothelioma such as synovial sarcoma and thymic epithelial tumor (Fig. 12-6). Further,

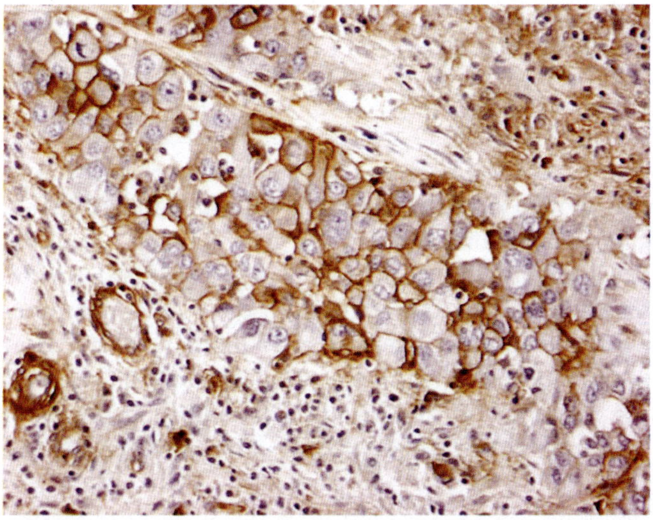

FIGURE 12-5: Thrombomodulin expression in diffuse malignant mesothelioma, showing delicate membranous expression. Note vascular endothelial staining at lower left.

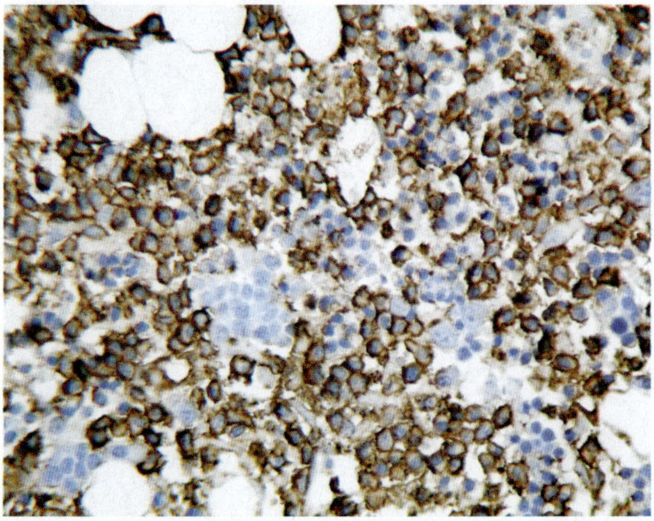

FIGURE 12-6: Thrombomodulin expression in thymic epithelial tumor.

granular cytoplasmic expression of thrombomodulin may be observed in adenocarcinomas and in some diffuse malignant mesotheliomas, particularly in areas associated with cellular degeneration and necrosis.

Epithelial Membrane Antigen

Epithelial membrane antigen (EMA) is expressed in both epithelioid diffuse malignant mesothelioma and in carcinomas, but their patterns of immunolocalization differ. EMA staining shows a membranous pattern with little or no cytoplasmic expression in diffuse malignant mesothelioma (Fig. 12-7). In contrast, EMA staining in carcinomas is predominantly cytoplasmic and membranous. This same staining distribution occurs with HMBE1 antibody. As discussed below, EMA is an important marker in helping distinguish reactive mesothelial cell proliferations (which are generally negative) from neoplastic mesothelial proliferations (which are generally positive). It is important to recognize that EMA may be expressed in a wide variety of tissues and cells including plasma cells, macrophages/histiocytes, melanoma, epithelioid vascular sarcoma, and some anaplastic large cell lymphomas, all of which show cytoplasmic expression.

Mesothelin (MSLN)

Mesothelin is a 40-kDa protein present in normal and neoplastic mesothelial cells and several tumors including ovarian and pancreatic adenocarcinoma. The precise biologic function of mesothelin is not known although the protein may be involved in cell adhesion. OVCAR-3, an ovarian tumor cell line, was initially used as immunogen for the generation of the murine monoclonal antibody K1. This later became the antimesothelin monoclonal antibody. In one study, K1 was found to have high sensitivity and specificity for diffuse malignant mesothelioma in all 19 diffuse malignant mesotheliomas (15 epithelioid and 4 biphasic subtypes), in contrast to 0/23 (0%) of lung adenocarcinomas.[25] Subsequently Ordonez in 2003 reported mesothelin expression in 100% of 44 epithelioid diffuse malignant mesotheliomas and no expression in 8 sarcomatoid diffuse malignant mesotheliomas.[26] Mesothelin was found to be

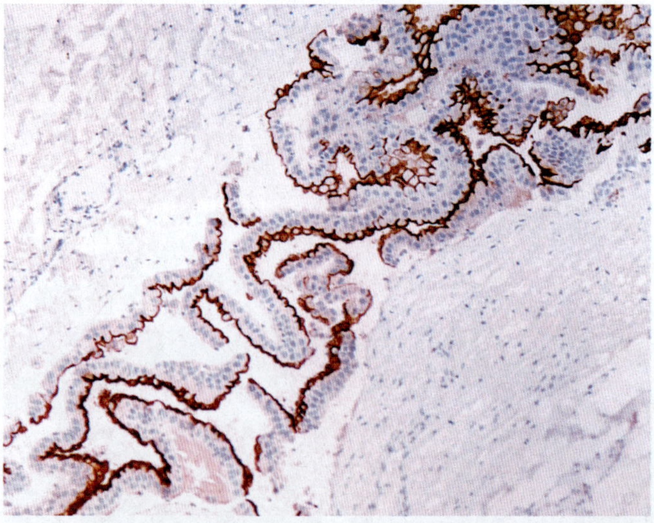

FIGURE 12-7: Epithelial membrane antigen staining of epithelioid mesothelium, showing membranous expression.

expressed in ovarian and peritoneal adenocarcinoma (100%), pancreatic adenocarcinoma (91%), endometrial adenocarcinoma (67%), gastric adenocarcinoma (50%), and colonic adenocarcinoma (31%). 3/17 (18%) of squamous carcinomas of the lung were also noted to be weakly positive. There was no expression of mesothelin in the breast, renal, thyroid, or prostatic carcinomas tested. Overall, mesothelin has high sensitivity in epithelioid diffuse malignant mesothelioma but limited use in sarcomatoid mesothelioma.

Calretinin

Calretinin is a calcium-binding protein of 29 kDa belonging to the troponin C family. Calretinin plays a role in diverse cellular functions including intracellular calcium buffering, messaging, and modulating neuronal excitability and as a diagnostic marker in some cancers and diseases including Hirschsprung disease. Calretinin stains normal and neoplastic mesothelial cells and has been extensively studied to help differentiate these from lung tumors (Table 12-10). Calretinin expression is observed in over 90% of epithelioid diffuse malignant mesotheliomas with more specificity recognized when both nuclear and cytoplasmic stainings are observed (Fig. 12-8). Calretinin expression is also observed in approximately 45% of sarcomatoid diffuse malignant mesotheliomas, although expression is of lower intensity and focal in nature. Calretinin is expressed in both normal and neoplastic mesothelial cells and has no role in distinguishing benign from malignant mesothelium.[10,14,27–31]

Calretinin is regarded as a first-line positive mesothelial marker in distinguishing epithelioid diffuse malignant mesothelioma from adenocarcinoma and has a role, albeit more limited, in the positive identification of sarcomatoid diffuse malignant mesothelioma (Fig. 12-9). It is recognized that calretinin expression can be found in some adenocarcinomas, particularly giant cell carcinomas, as well as synovial sarcoma (Fig. 12-10). Such immunoreactivity may provide significant challenges to the surgical pathologist. In such cases, it is important to consider the gross tumor distribution. Diffuse malignant mesothelioma is typically a diffuse serosal tumor, whereas lung carcinomas and sarcomas often form masses. In distinguishing synovial sarcoma, it is helpful to obtain cytogenetic testing for the X:18 translocation, which is present in over 95% of synovial sarcomas and absent in diffuse malignant mesothelioma. A meta-analysis by King of 17 studies, consisting of 885 epithelioid diffuse malignant mesotheliomas and 912 pulmonary adenocarcinomas, reported calretinin sensitivity of 82% and specificity of 85% for epithelioid diffuse malignant mesothelioma.[2]

Table 12-10 Calretinin expression in epithelioid diffuse malignant mesothelioma

Author	Diffuse Malignant Mesothelioma	Carcinomas
Doglioni et al.[27]	44/44 (100%)	28/294 (9.5%)
Ordonez[10]	38/38 (100%)	3/38 (8%)
Ordonez[28]	42/42 (100%)	2/23 (9%)
Barberis et al.[29]	8/8 (100%)	3/13 (23%)
Brockstedt et al.[30]	110/119 (92%)	16/57 (28%)
Carella et al.[31]	40/46 (87%)	2/20 (10%)
Cury et al.[14]	47/51 (92%)	1/59 (2%)

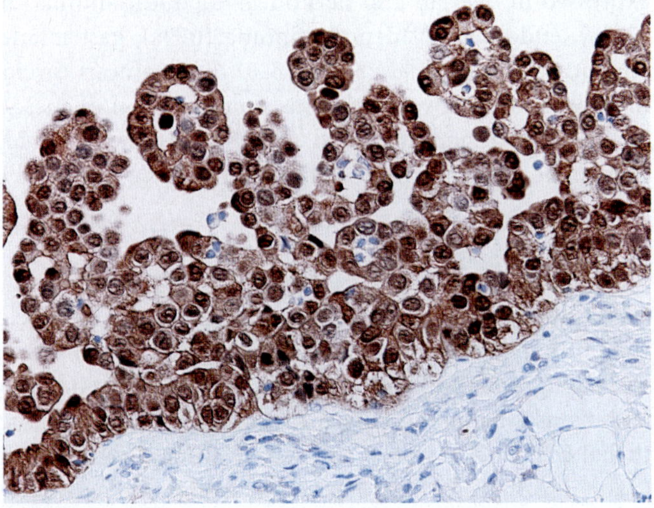

FIGURE 12-8: Calretinin staining, with both nuclear and cytoplasmic expression, in epithelioid diffuse malignant mesothelioma.

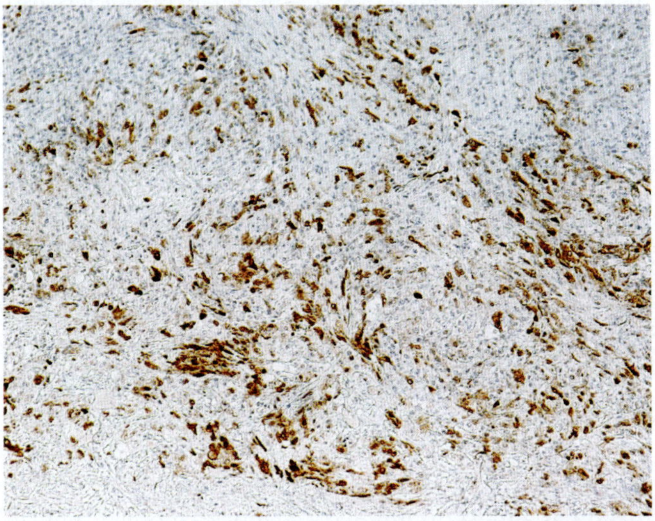

FIGURE 12-9: Calretinin expression in sarcomatoid diffuse malignant mesothelioma, showing only focal expression.

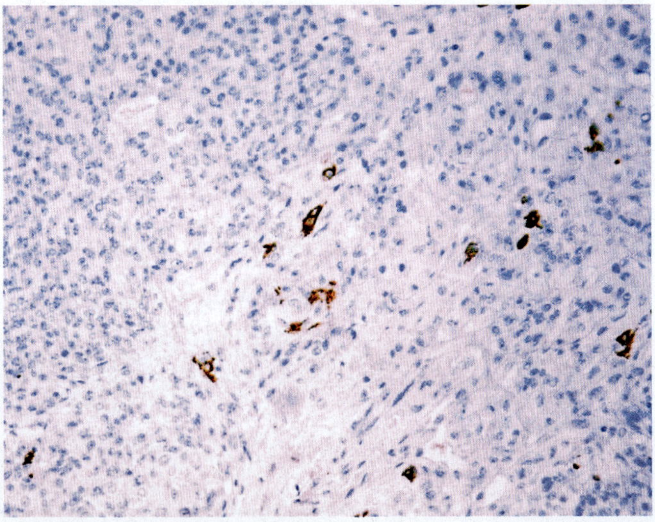

FIGURE 12-10: Calretinin expression in synovial sarcoma.

Calretinin is commercially available in polyclonal (Swant, Chemicon, Zymed) antisera with reported improved sensitivity and specificity from Zymed antibody against human recombinant calretinin.

Some metastatic carcinomas principally RCCs and colonic adenocarcinomas (particularly poorly differentiated forms) may be calretinin positive. There has been focus comparing epithelioid diffuse malignant mesothelioma with pulmonary adenocarcinoma, with few studies examining calretinin expression in lung cancer by histologic subtype. Calretinin expression has been observed in well-differentiated acinar-type pulmonary adenocarcinomas (11%); large cell carcinoma, not otherwise specified (38%); large cell neuroendocrine carcinoma (45%); small cell carcinoma (49%); squamous cell carcinoma (34%); and giant cell carcinoma (67%).[32] Ironically, one potential pitfall is the overall popularity of calretinin; it is often the first immunostain considered by the surgical pathologist, who then might give too much weight to its positivity or negativity in an individual case, without appropriate regard to the entire immunostain panel. Another potential pitfall is overinterpretation by the surgical pathologist of a calretinin stain of poor technical quality.

Podoplanin (D2-40)

Podoplanin (D2-40) is a 38-kDa transmembrane glycoprotein expressed in kidney podocytes, skeletal and myocardial muscle, placenta, osteoblasts, lymphatic endothelium, and reactive and neoplastic mesothelial cells. The physiologic function of podoplanin is not known although it is recognized that its expression is up-regulated in different human cancers including diffuse malignant mesothelioma, head and neck squamous carcinomas, and many tumors in the central nervous system. Podoplanin expression is mainly detected in squamous cell carcinomas, central nervous system tumors, germ cell neoplasia, and diffuse malignant mesothelioma.[33–36] (Fig. 12-11) (Table 12-11). D2-40 monoclonal antibody was raised against M2a protein derived from germ cell tumors.

D2-40 is a useful positive mesothelial marker in distinguishing epithelioid diffuse malignant mesothelioma from lung adenocarcinoma. For sarcomatoid diffuse malignant mesothelioma, the literature is conflicting. Potential interpretive pitfalls exist as podoplanin is constantly expressed in lymphatic endothelium and serves as an internal positive control

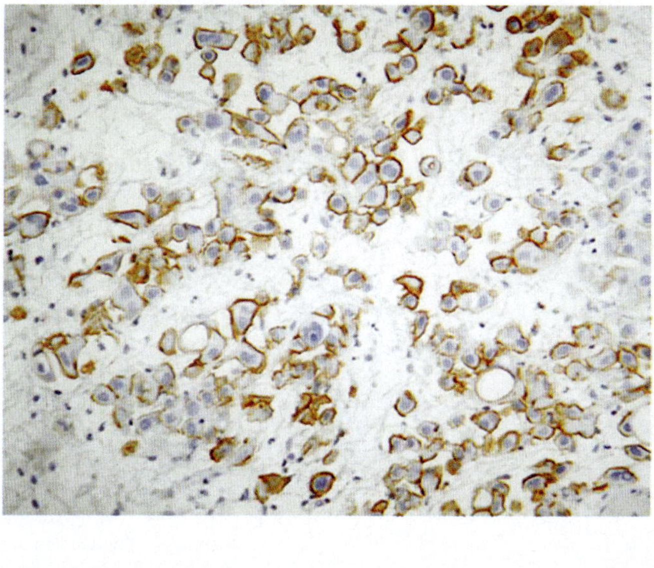

FIGURE 12-11: D2-40 (podoplanin) staining in epithelioid diffuse malignant mesothelioma, showing membranous expression.

Table 12-11 D2-40 expression in diffuse malignant mesothelioma

Author	Diffuse Malignant Mesothelioma	Carcinomas
Kimura[33]	5/5 (100%)	0/93 (0%)
Ordonez[34]	28/30 (93%)	ND[a]
Chu et al.[35]	51/53 (96%)	0/30 (0%)
Ordonez[36]	25/29 (86%)	0/34 (0%)

[a]ND, not done.

in tissues. It is important that the surgical pathologist does not overinterpret focal linear membrane expression within lymphatics. D2-40 may serve as a useful marker in distinguishing epithelioid diffuse malignant mesothelioma from squamous cell carcinoma (where cytokeratin 5/6 and thrombomodulin have no utility). D2-40 is expressed in malignant vascular sarcomas in the pleura. If malignant epithelioid vascular sarcoma is considered, CD31 and CD34 immunostaining should be performed, as these are not expressed in diffuse malignant mesothelioma. Subserosal spindle cells may label with D2-40, so care should be exercised in interpreting these areas (Fig. 12-12).

Wilms Tumor 1 Susceptibility Gene

Wilms tumor 1 susceptibility (WT1) gene encodes a transcription factor that has an essential role in the development of the urogenital system. WT1 protein has a host of cellular factors. It is expressed in infantile renal tissue and Wilms tumors and in adults in the ovary and testis and in normal and neoplastic mesothelium. It is a positive mesothelial marker in epithelioid diffuse malignant mesothelioma in discriminating it from adenocarcinoma.[37–39] In a meta-analysis by King, WT1 product was found to have 77% sensitivity and 96% specificity for

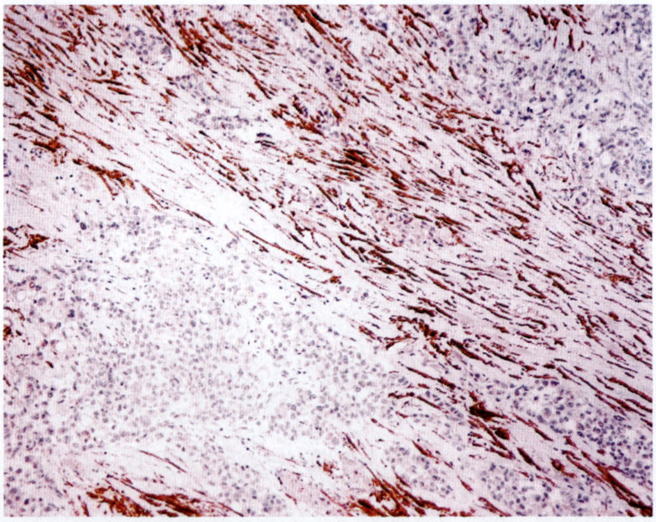

FIGURE 12-12: D2-40 expression in reactive subserosal spindle cells. Note the area of negative tumor staining, a potential pitfall.

Table 12-12 WT1 expression in diffuse malignant mesothelioma

Author	Diffuse Malignant Mesothelioma	Carcinomas
Amin et al.[37]	20/21 (95%)	0/20 (0%)
Foster et al.[38]	50/67 (75%)	0/51 (0%)
Ordonez[39]	28/30 (93%)	ND[a]

[a]Not done.

epithelioid diffuse malignant mesothelioma[2] (Table 12-12). The meta-analysis review of eight studies, consisting of 264 epithelioid diffuse malignant mesotheliomas and 213 pulmonary adenocarcinomas, reported 77% sensitivity and 96% specificity of WT1 for diffuse malignant mesothelioma. It is important to focus on nuclear expression, as cytoplasmic expression alone is nonspecific (Fig. 12-13). WT1 may be expressed in endothelium, and an awareness of this is important to prevent misdiagnosis.

WT1 is a useful positive marker in distinguishing epithelioid diffuse malignant mesothelioma from adenocarcinoma when there is nuclear WT1 expression (Fig. 12-14). WT1 has limited utility as a positive marker of sarcomatoid diffuse malignant mesothelioma. WT1 is not the preferred positive mesothelial marker for peritoneal tumors, especially in females, due to its constant expression in serous ovarian carcinomas.

HBME1

HBME1 is the monoclonal antibody generated from an epithelioid diffuse malignant mesothelioma cell line. The antibody shows thick membrane expression in epithelioid diffuse malignant mesothelioma. It is useful in distinguishing epithelioid diffuse malignant mesothelioma from adenocarcinoma, where a fine, thin membrane and cytoplasmic expression

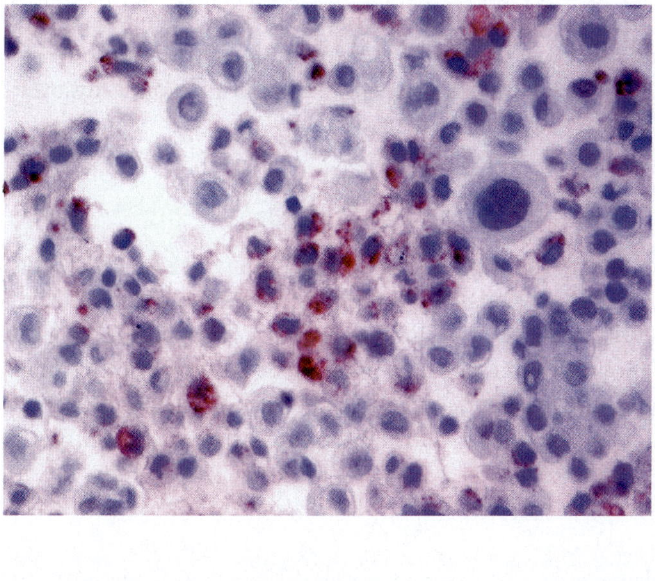

FIGURE 12-13: Nonspecific expression of WT1 in diffuse malignant mesothelioma, showing cytoplasmic granular deposition.

FIGURE 12-14: Nuclear WT1 in diffuse malignant mesothelioma.

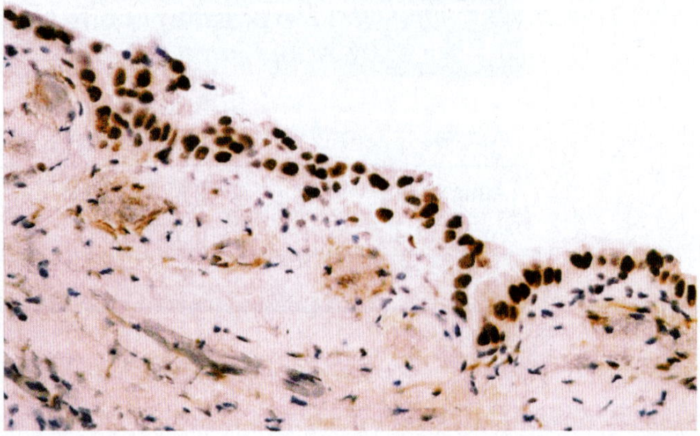

occurs, although many investigators no longer champion the use of this marker in the presence of other more robustly validated positive mesothelial markers. HBME1 has no utility in the positive identification of sarcomatoid diffuse malignant mesothelioma. HMBE1 is also expressed in carcinoma, chordoma, and follicular and papillary carcinoma of the thyroid. A meta-analysis review of 14 studies, consisting of 769 epithelioid diffuse malignant mesotheliomas and 676 pulmonary adenocarcinomas, reported 85% sensitivity and 43% specificity of HBME1 for epithelioid diffuse malignant mesothelioma.[2]

EMERGING NOVEL MARKERS USED TO DISTINGUISH MALIGNANT EPITHELIOID TUMORS

Caveolin-1

Caveolin-1 is a 22-kDa transmembrane protein expressed in a variety of mesenchymal cells including endothelial cells, smooth muscle cells, type 1 and type 2 pneumocytes, and mesothelial cells. Caveolin-1 is commonly up-regulated in a variety of malignant neoplasms and has been reported to have a role in tumor progression and drug resistance in advanced non–small cell lung cancer.[40] In lung carcinomas, staining is predominantly membranous in nature. Caveolin-1 has been reported to be positive in epithelioid diffuse malignant mesothelioma with 100% sensitivity and 93% specificity.[41]

Napsin A

Napsin A is an aspartic proteinase of approximately 38 kDa expressed in type 2 pneumocytes, in alveolar macrophages, and in the kidney. Napsin A expression is within the cytoplasm, and it has been reported to be a useful marker for primary lung adenocarcinoma. It has been reported in between 77% and 93% of cases with little expression in other nonpulmonary adenocarcinomas or other histologic subtypes of lung cancer. There has been no reported napsin A expression in diffuse malignant mesothelioma. Napsin expression was identified in 49/118 (42%) of RCCs.[42,43]

Tenascin

The tenascin family comprises four extracellular matrix glycoproteins termed tenascin C, tenascin X, tenascin R, and tenascin W of over 300 kDa. Tenascins modulate cell matrix interactions by means of intracellular P38 map kinase pathways and mediate cell motility. Tenascin X has been reported to be a novel diagnostic marker of diffuse malignant mesothelioma expressed in 33/36 (92%) diffuse malignant mesotheliomas compared with 5/47 (11%) ovarian carcinomas/primary peritoneal carcinomas.[44] Tenascin X was detected in only 2/12 (17%) lung carcinomas (in effusions) with <5% cells positive. Tenascin X was also found to be predominantly negative in reactive mesothelial proliferations.[44]

Osteopontin

Osteopontin is a 32-kDa integrin cell adhesion molecule mediating cell matrix adhesions and binding CD44. Osteopontin has been reported to be expressed in all subtypes of diffuse malignant mesothelioma. It is also expressed in various carcinomas, including lung carcinoma, and is associated with tumor progression and poor prognosis. Osteopontin has been reported in 36/28 (95%) diffuse malignant mesotheliomas and in 12/17 (71%) lung carcinomas. Serum osteopontin levels have been reported to be higher in patients with asbestos-related diffuse malignant mesotheliomas than those without asbestos exposure; however, this claim has not been validated.[45]

PAX 8

Paired box 8 (PAX 8) is oncodevelopmental transcription gene involved in cell differentiation. PAX 8 has been reported to be positive in serous ovarian carcinomas and negative in 24 pleural and 23 peritoneal diffuse malignant mesotheliomas (however, all but 3 were of epithelioid subtype).[46]

OTHER POSITIVE MESOTHELIAL MARKERS

The literature contains various putative positive mesothelial markers, and these are briefly listed in this section. None has consistently stood the test of time and none is now recommended for diagnostic purposes. These markers include AMAD-1 and AMAD-2 (Donna antibody), parathyroid hormone–like peptide, ME1 and ME2, and MS 1.

LOGISTIC REGRESSION METHODOLOGIES

Due to the recognized plasticity of mesothelium, and tumor diversity in diffuse malignant mesothelioma, it is recognized that an appropriate selection of antibodies is a critical step in optimizing the diagnosis of diffuse malignant mesothelioma. There exist limitations to meta-analytical studies on account of interlaboratory variability and antisera clone selection. More recent studies have focused on logistic regression methodologies to optimize the diagnosis of epithelioid diffuse malignant mesothelioma and its distinction from pulmonary adenocarcinoma. Maximal sensitivity (over 96%) and specificity have been obtained by means of a three-antibody panel consisting of calretinin, BG8, and MOC-31.[47] Bayesian statistical analysis of the previously published meta-analytical studies found that selected antibodies, either single or in pairs, were at least as effective as more extensive panels in distinguishing diffuse malignant mesothelioma from metastatic pulmonary adenocarcinoma.[48] The incorporation of TTF-1 with WT1 was found to represent the best evidence-based choice of immunomarkers to confirm diffuse malignant mesothelioma. More recently, by tree-based regression analysis, to define the minimal set of antibodies for identifying diffuse malignant mesothelioma, a positive reactivity with calretinin coupled with BG8 negativity was regarded as highly predictive of definite diffuse malignant mesothelioma.[49]

ROLE OF IMMUNOHISTOCHEMISTRY IN NEOPLASTIC SPINDLE CELL TUMORS OF THE SEROSA

General immunohistochemistry is limited in its utility to separate spindle cell tumors arising in the serosa although it does contribute to allowing for a confident diagnosis of diffuse malignant mesothelioma.

Cytokeratin has the most important role in differentiating sarcomatoid diffuse malignant mesotheliomas (which are positive) from most sarcomas (which are negative). In general, nonmesothelial spindle cell proliferations, reactive or neoplastic, are cytokeratin negative. Cytokeratin positivity in a diffuse serosal-based tumor with spindle cell morphology clearly favors a diagnosis of sarcomatoid diffuse malignant mesothelioma over sarcoma. However, there are pitfalls. First, it is recognized that not all sarcomatoid diffuse malignant mesotheliomas are cytokeratin positive, and second, some bona fide malignant sarcomas, most notably those with epithelioid characteristics, are known to express cytokeratin. These include leiomyosarcoma, epithelioid vascular sarcomas, and synovial sarcoma.

It is recognized that submesothelial spindled cells express low molecular weight cytokeratin, and these may undergo proliferative changes in a variety of inflammatory conditions, which may prompt the unwary pathologist to overdiagnose sarcomatoid diffuse malignant mesothelioma. The cellular distribution of cytokeratin expression is useful in separating benign from neoplastic mesothelial proliferations (Fig. 12-15).

The mesothelial markers have more limited utility in identifying sarcomatoid diffuse malignant mesothelioma and other spindle cell malignancies (Table 12-13). It has been

FIGURE 12-15: Cytokeratin staining in reactive cellular pleuritis, showing parallel linear expression without disarray.

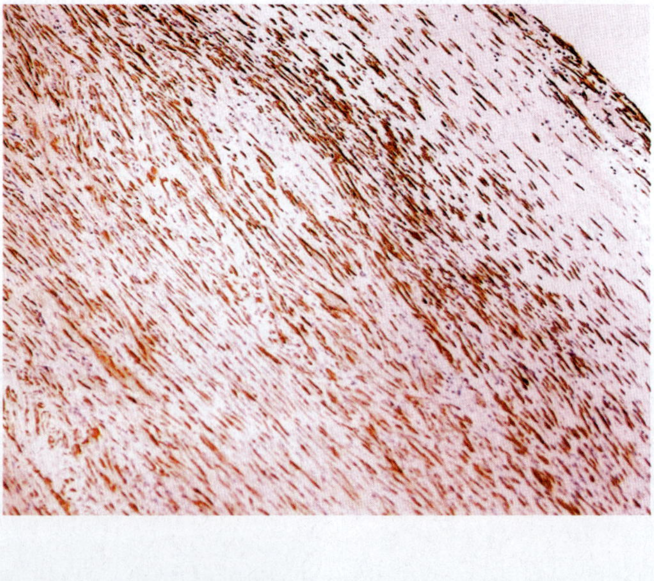

Table 12-13 Mesothelial markers in sarcomatoid diffuse malignant mesothelioma

Mesothelioma Immunohistochemistry					
Meso Sarcoma SPCA	**CK**	**Calret**	**CK 5/6**	**Thr**	**WT1**
Cardiff	**77**	**39**	**29**	**29**	—
(*n* = 31 MES)	32	0	4	16	
(*n* = 30 SAR)	100	0	0	0	
(*n* = 4 SPCA)					
Lucas	**83**	**70**	**0**	**60**	**0**
(*n* = 20 MES)	17	17	0	38	4
	100	60	4	40	0
Doglioni	**100**	**100**	—	—	—
(*n* = 3 MES)					
Oates	**100**	—	**50**	—	—
(*n* = 8 MES)					

proposed that podoplanin (D2-40) is a useful marker for the diagnosis of sarcomatoid diffuse malignant mesothelioma; however, this requires further validation.

In the differential diagnosis of spindle cell tumors of the pleura, it is important to consider the anatomical tumor distribution, that is, a diffuse pleural-based tumor composed of cytokeratin-positive spindle cells strongly favors diffuse malignant mesothelioma over metastatic sarcomatoid carcinoma or sarcoma. Sarcomatoid carcinomas are usually more localized mass lesions. The neoplastic spindle cells will be cytokeratin positive, and there may be other areas of differentiation, most likely squamous or glandular components, less likely neuroendocrine differentiation. In some cases, there will be focal expression of the carcinoma markers. The most robust means of distinguishing sarcomatoid diffuse malignant mesothelioma from sarcomatoid carcinoma is in the differences in the gross anatomical distribution of the tumors. Most sarcomas are cytokeratin negative. The differential diagnosis of malignant spindle cell tumors of the pleura includes sarcomatoid diffuse malignant mesothelioma, sarcomatoid carcinoma and, sarcoma. The role of immunohistochemistry in this setting to positively identify diffuse malignant mesothelioma relies predominantly on the demonstration of keratin positivity within the spindle cells and, to a lesser extent, expression of the positive mesothelial markers. Broad-spectrum cytokeratins (AE1/3), CAM 5.2 (cytokeratins 8 and 18), and MNF 116 may be used singly or preferably in concert to optimize the localization of keratin positivity. Most sarcomatoid diffuse malignant mesotheliomas and sarcomatoid carcinomas show relatively strong and diffuse expression with cytokeratins. The keratin cocktail of AE1/AE3/CAM 5.2 and MNF 116 identified immunoreactivity in 93% of 280 sarcomatoid diffuse malignant mesothelioma cases in one large series.[50] This contrasts with most sarcomas although exceptions exist. It is now recognized that many sarcomas have epithelioid morphologic variants and these may express cytokeratin, especially CAM 5.2. In general, when cytokeratin expression is observed in sarcomas, it is of low intensity and focal. However, with synovial sarcoma, cytokeratin expression may also be strong and diffuse.

The differential diagnosis between sarcomatoid diffuse malignant mesothelioma and synovial sarcoma is particularly challenging. Certain morphologic similarities exist, and, in addition, immunophenotypic similarities are present. First, synovial sarcomas may show cytokeratin positivity and, in addition, may express the mesothelial markers calretinin, CK5/6, and thrombomodulin. Most synovial sarcomas are localized tumors, and definitive distinction from diffuse malignant mesothelioma may be made by cytogenetic analysis and confirmation of the X:18 translocation present in over 96% of synovial sarcomas, but absent in diffuse malignant mesothelioma.

It is recognized that malignant solitary fibrous tumor, desmoid tumor, and pleural thymoma (WHO type A) may closely mimic diffuse malignant mesothelioma. For malignant solitary fibrous tumor, cytokeratin expression is not seen and the tumors show CD34, Bcl-2, and CD99 expression. For pleural desmoid tumors, again cytokeratin is negative and there is observed expression of smooth muscle actin, desmin, and β catenin. Primary pleural thymomas of WHO type A have a spindle cell morphology and these will typically be cytokeratin positive. Additionally they have been reported to express cytokeratin 5/6 and thrombomodulin. Calretinin is typically negative in the tumor cells, although stromal mast cells will be calretinin positive.

ROLE OF IMMUNOHISTOCHEMISTRY IN SEPARATING REACTIVE FROM NEOPLASTIC MESOTHELIAL PROLIFERATIONS

Reactive mesothelial proliferations may be either epithelioid or composed of cellular spindle cells. In each case the differential diagnosis differs. On the one hand reactive mesothelial proliferations of epithelioid type must be distinguished from malignant epithelioid proliferations. In contrast, reactive spindle cell proliferations must be distinguished from malignant spindle cell tumors, in particular desmoplastic diffuse malignant mesothelioma. Benign versus malignant dilemmas exist particularly in small biopsy specimens. Immunohistochemistry is of more use distinguishing reactive from neoplastic epithelioid mesothelial proliferations than it is for spindle cell lesions.

A number of markers have been tested, although the most reliable markers in this setting are EMA and p53 (both preferentially expressed in neoplastic mesothelium) combined with desmin (preferentially expressed in reactive mesothelium).

Epithelial Membrane Antigen

EMA is a high molecular weight transmembrane glycoprotein found in human milk fat globule membranes. EMA is identified in most normal and neoplastic epithelial settings (usually with cytoplasmic elaboration) and is also seen in plasma cells, activated B lymphocytes, diffuse malignant mesotheliomas (membranous elaboration), mesenchymal tissues, and some lymphomas (anaplastic large cell lymphoma). EMA has been studied in relation to separating adenocarcinoma from epithelioid diffuse malignant mesothelioma on the basis of cellular localization (cytoplasmic versus membranous), although most investigators do not advocate use of the marker for this purpose.

EMA is a first-line marker in distinguishing reactive (benign) mesothelial proliferations from diffuse malignant mesothelioma.[51,52] Interpretive problems may exist when there is only focal low-intensity expression, which may be seen in benign proliferations. As a consequence, it is important not to overinterpret focal EMA expression. Instead, consider the pathology in light of other useful markers (such as P53 and desmin) and the clinicoradiologic and other pathologic findings. Reactive mesothelium is usually EMA negative (Table 12-14).

Table 12-14 EMA expression in reactive and neoplastic mesothelial proliferations

Marker	Reactive Hyperplasia	Diffuse Malignant Mesothelioma	Author
EMA (clone Mc5)	12/20 (60%)	14/20 (70%)	Saad[51]
EMA (clone E29)	0/20 (0%)	15/20 (75%)	Saad[51]
EMA (clone E29)	8/40 (20%)	48/60 (80%)	Attanoos[52]

P53

P53 is a tumor suppressor gene located on the short arm of chromosome 17, which encodes a 53-kDa nuclear phosphoprotein involved in transcription regulation and cell growth. P53 mutations are common in human neoplasia and are noted in diffuse malignant mesotheliomas but not in reactive mesothelial proliferations. P53 immunostaining requires appropriate antigen retrieval, preferably by microwave heating. P53 expression is seen in about one-third of lung carcinomas. Nuclear P53 expression may be patchy particularly in cytologic preparations (Fig. 12-16).

Desmin

Desmin is an intermediate filament found in smooth cardiac and striated muscle and in a variety of mesenchymal tumors including those of muscle origin. Desmin has been reported in diffuse malignant mesotheliomas (with leiomyoid differentiation). Reactive mesothelial cells are positive for desmin, in contrast to most epithelioid diffuse malignant mesotheliomas and carcinomas, which are negative.[16,52–54] This is useful in both serous cytology effusions and histologic specimens (Table 12-15).

A number of other markers have been tested in reactive mesothelium and diffuse malignant mesothelioma, including Bcl-2, P-glycoprotein, (P170), platelet-derived growth factor receptor β chain, rep 86, and GLUT1.

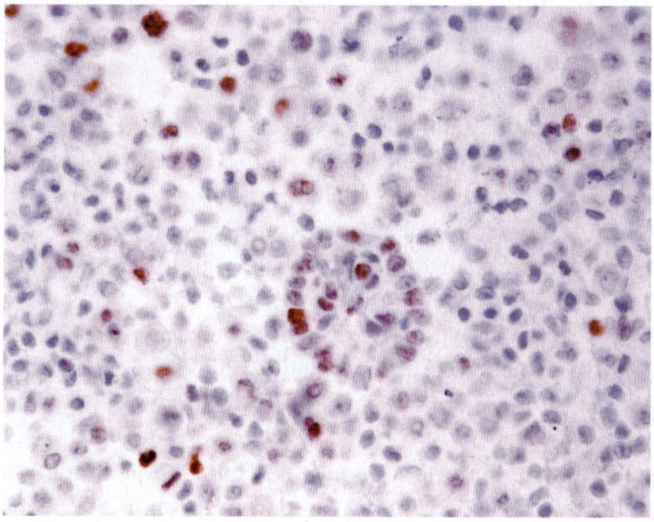

FIGURE 12-16: Patchy p53 staining in a cytologic preparation; a final diagnosis of diffuse malignant mesothelioma was rendered on biopsy.

Table 12-15 Desmin expression in reactive and neoplastic mesothelial proliferations

Antibody	Reactive Mesothelial Hyperplasia	Diffuse Malignant Mesothelioma	Author
Desmin	34/40 (85%)	6/60 (10%)	Attanoos et al.[52]
Desmin	47/56 (84%)	1/12 (8%)	Davidson et al.[53]
	+	ND	Kupryjaczyka[54]
	ND[a]	9/16 (56%)	Mayall et al.[16]

[a]ND, not done.

Glut 1

Glut 1 is a member of a glucose transporter family. Glut 1 has limited expression in normal tissues being present in erythrocytes, renal tubules, placenta, testicular germinal cells, and perineurium. Glut 1 is expressed in a range of carcinomas (breast, lung, head and neck, bladder, and renal cell) and is strongly expressed in colorectal carcinomas. Glut 1 has been reported to be positive in diffuse malignant mesothelioma and show limited expression in reactive effusions. Kato reported expression in 40/40 (100%) diffuse malignant mesotheliomas with no expression seen in 40 (0%) benign mesothelial proliferations.[55] Glut 1 appears to have a very limited role in positively marking sarcomatoid diffuse malignant mesothelioma.

A number of proliferation markers that include MCM-2 and Ki-67 have been studied and appear of limited value.

REACTIVE VERSUS NEOPLASTIC SPINDLE CELL LESIONS

Immunohistochemistry has little value in the distinction between benign spindle cell proliferation and sarcomatoid diffuse malignant mesothelioma. Keratin is useful in facilitating the identification of subtle areas of mesothelial cell invasion at the advancing tumor edge. In a minority of malignant mesotheliomas, P53 and EMA may be expressed; however, in this setting, the markers have low sensitivity, and therefore, negative staining is of limited value.

Human Telomerase Reverse Transcriptase

Telomerase is a polymerase enzyme, which adds telomeric DNA sequences to the ends of chromosomes and is required to stain cell division. Telomerase is not present in normal somatic cells but is identified in stem cells, germ cells, and malignant cells. The presence of telomerase can be demonstrated by immunohistochemistry with nuclear and cytoplasmic expression. Telomerase activity has been identified in approximately 85% of human cancers. It has been proposed as a marker to distinguish benign mesothelial proliferations from diffuse malignant mesothelioma. Telomerase activity was demonstrated in 67/68 (99%) malignant mesotheliomas and in 0/3 (0%) of benign mesothelial proliferations.[56] Further studies are required to validate the utility of this marker in distinguishing reactive from neoplastic mesothelial proliferations.

Table 12-16 contains a summary of common immunopanels; and Table 12-17 contains a summary of the benefits and limitations of certain commonly used immunostains.

Table 12-16 Summary of common immunopanels

A. Epithelioid diffuse malignant mesothelioma/lung adenocarcinoma	
Calretinin	TTF-1
Cytokeratin 5/6	MOC-31
WT1	BG8
D2-40	CEA
B. Epithelioid diffuse malignant mesothelioma/squamous carcinoma	
WT1	p63 (p40)
Calretinin	MOC-31
	BG8
(No use: cytokeratin 5/6, thrombomodulin, D2-40)	
C. Epithelioid diffuse malignant mesothelioma/RCC clear cell variant	
Cytokeratin 5/6	Leu M1
Calretinin	RCC
Mesothelin	
(No use: CEA, BG8, Ber EP4, thrombomodulin, WT1)	
D. Peritoneal epithelioid diffuse malignant mesothelioma/serous carcinoma	
Calretinin	MOC31
D2-40	BG8
(No use: CK 5/6, WT1, CEA)	

Table 12-17 Benefits and limitations of certain commonly used immunostains

Carcinoembryonic Antigen (CEA)

Benefits: Polyclonal CEA has high specificity for adenocarcinoma and is widely regarded as a first-line marker of adenocarcinoma and very useful in distinguishing the tumor from pleural diffuse malignant mesothelioma.

Limitations: False-positive reactions exist with nonspecific antigen staining. Polyclonal CEA may label hyaluronate-rich epithelioid diffuse malignant mesotheliomas. Pretreatment with hyaluronidase prior to immunohistochemical staining reduces this false-positive staining. These are so-called "mucin-positive" epithelioid diffuse malignant mesotheliomas. CEA is typically negative in RCC and serous papillary ovarian carcinomas, limiting its use in distinguishing diffuse malignant mesothelioma from adenocarcinoma in the peritoneum.

Leu M1 (CD15)

Benefits: Leu M1 is a very useful marker for distinguishing adenocarcinoma from epithelioid diffuse malignant mesothelioma.

Limitations: Leu M1 staining may be focal and problematic to interpret due to the presence of positive inflammatory cells and necrotic regions in small biopsies.

Ber EP4

Benefits: Ber EP4 is a useful marker in distinguishing adenocarcinoma from diffuse malignant mesothelioma.

Limitations: Adenocarcinomas usually show a predominantly circumferential membranous staining pattern with up to 20% of diffuse malignant mesotheliomas showing focal expression, usually with lateral membrane staining.

(Continued)

Table 12-17 Benefits and limitations of certain commonly used immunostains *(Continued)*

TTF-1

Benefits: TTF-1 is a very useful first-line positive epithelial marker of pulmonary adenocarcinoma and small cell carcinoma. There are no reported cases of TTF-1 expressed in diffuse malignant mesothelioma. TTF-1 is useful in predicting whether a small cell carcinoma is of pulmonary (positive) or extrapulmonary (negative) origin.

Pancytokeratin

Benefits: Pankeratin markers have very limited use as discriminating markers of epithelioid diffuse malignant mesothelioma and adenocarcinoma. Also, for malignant epithelioid tumors in the pleura, pancytokeratin negativity strongly militates against the diagnosis of bona fide diffuse malignant mesothelioma and metastatic carcinoma. Alternate diagnoses such as epithelioid variant sarcomas, most notably epithelioid vascular sarcomas (epithelioid hemangioendothelioma or epithelioid angiosarcoma), malignant melanoma, or lymphoma, should be considered.

Cell Adhesion Molecules

Limitations: Not advocated as a first-line marker for diffuse malignant mesothelioma (N-cadherin) or adenocarcinoma (E-cadherin), although both have utility as complimentary second-line markers

Thrombomodulin

Benefits: Thrombomodulin is best regarded as a second-line mesothelial marker because of its relatively low sensitivity for epithelioid diffuse malignant mesothelioma and very limited utility in sarcomatoid diffuse malignant mesothelioma. However, there is evidence thrombomodulin may be preferentially expressed in small cell diffuse malignant mesothelioma. It usually shows prominent membranous expression.

Limitations: Interpretive problems exist with thrombomodulin due to its expression in endothelium. Focal linear and noncircumferential thrombomodulin staining may be overinterpreted as positive, especially in potential sarcomatoid diffuse malignant mesothelioma cases. The same interpretive problem is encountered with D2-40 (podoplanin). Thrombomodulin (together with cytokeratin 5/6) is typically expressed in squamous epithelial cells and its tumors, urothelial cells and its tumors, and in selected tumors, which may mimic diffuse malignant mesothelioma such as synovial sarcoma and thymic epithelial tumor. Granular cytoplasmic expression of thrombomodulin may be observed in adenocarcinomas and in some diffuse malignant mesotheliomas, particularly in areas associated with cellular degeneration and necrosis.

Calretinin

Benefits: Calretinin is regarded as a first-line positive mesothelial marker in distinguishing epithelioid diffuse malignant mesothelioma from adenocarcinoma and has a role, albeit more limited, in the positive identification of sarcomatoid diffuse malignant mesothelioma.

Limitations: Some metastatic carcinomas, principally RCCs and colonic adenocarcinomas (particularly poorly differentiated forms), may be calretinin positive. Calretinin expression has been observed in well-differentiated acinar-type pulmonary adenocarcinomas; large cell carcinoma, not otherwise specified; large cell neuroendocrine carcinoma; small cell carcinoma; squamous cell carcinoma; and giant cell carcinoma.

Podoplanin (D2-40)

Benefits: D2-40 is a useful positive mesothelial marker in distinguishing epithelioid diffuse malignant mesothelioma from lung adenocarcinoma. For sarcomatoid mesothelioma, the literature is conflicting.

Limitations: D2-40 is expressed in malignant vascular sarcomas in the pleura; if malignant epithelioid vascular sarcoma is considered, CD31 and CD34 immunostaining should be performed as this will not be expressed in diffuse malignant mesothelioma.

Table 12-17	Benefits and limitations of certain commonly used immunostains *(Continued)*

WT1

Benefits: This is a useful positive marker in distinguishing epithelioid diffuse malignant mesothelioma from adenocarcinoma.

Limitations: WT1 has limited utility as a positive marker of sarcomatoid diffuse malignant mesothelioma. WT1 is not the preferred positive mesothelial marker in the peritoneum, especially in females, due to its constant expression in serous ovarian carcinomas.

EMA

Benefits: EMA is a first-line marker in distinguishing reactive (benign) mesothelial proliferations (negative) from diffuse malignant mesothelioma (positive).

Limitations: Interpretive problems occur when there is only focal low-intensity expression, which may occur in benign proliferations.

References

1. Husain AN, Colby TV, Ordonez NG. Guidelines for pathologic diagnosis of malignant mesothelioma: a consensus statement from the International Mesothelioma Interest Group. *Arch Pathol Lab Med* 2009;133:1317–1331.
2. King JR, Thatcher N, Pickering CAC, et al. Sensitivity and specificity of immunohistochemical markers used in the diagnosis of epithelioid mesothelioma: a detailed systematic analysis using published data. *Histopathology* 2006;48:223–232.
3. Sheibani K, Battifora H, Burke JS. Antigenic phenotype of malignant mesotheliomas and pulmonary adenocarcinoma. An immunohistochemical analysis demonstrating the value of Leu M1 antigen. *Am J Pathol* 1986;123:212–219.
4. Otis CN, Carter D, Cole S, et al. Immunohistochemical evaluation of pleural mesothelioma and pulmonary adenocarcinoma. A bi-institutional study of 47 cases. *Am J Surg Pathol* 1987;11: 445–456.
5. Dejmek A, Hjerpe A. Carcinoembryonic antigen like reactivity in malignant mesothelioma. A comparison between different commercially available antibodies. *Cancer* 1994;73:464–469.
6. Bateman AC, al-Talib RK, Newman T, et al. Immunohistochemical phenotype of malignant mesothelioma: predictive value of CEA 125 and HBME 1 expression. *Histopathology* 1997;30:49–56.
7. Sheibani K, Esteban JM, Bailey A, et al. Immunologic and molecular studies as an aid to the diagnosis of malignant mesothelioma. *Hum Pathol* 1992;23:107–116.
8. Gaffey MJ, Mills FE, Swanson PE, et al. Immunoreactivity for Ber EP4 in adenocarcinoma, adenomatoid tumours and malignant mesotheliomas. *Am J Surg Pathol* 1992;16:593–599.
9. Dejmek A, Brockstedt U, Hjerpe A. Optimisation of a battery using 9 immunocytochemical variables for distinguishing between epithelial mesothelioma and adenocarcinoma. *APMIS* 1997;105:889–894.
10. Ordonez NG. Value of the Ber EP4 antibody in differentiating epithelial pleural mesothelium from adenocarcinoma. *Am J Clin Pathol* 1998;109:85–89.
11. Nagle RB. A review of intermediate filament biology and their use in pathological diagnosis. *Mol Biol Rep* 1994;19:3–21.
12. Moll R, Dhouailly D, Sun TT. Expression of cytokeratin 5. A distinctive feature of epithelial and biphasic mesotheliomas. *Virchows Arch B Cell Pathol Incl Mol Pathol* 1989;58:129–145.

13. Clover J, Oates J, Edwards C. Anticytokeratin 5/6: a positive marker for epithelioid mesothelioma. *Histopathology* 1997;31:140–143.
14. Cury PM, Butcher DN, Fisher C, et al. Mesothelium-associated antibodies thrombomodulin, cytokeratin 5/6, calretinin, and CD44H in distinguishing epithelioid pleural mesothelioma from adenocarcinoma metastatic to the pleura *Mod Pathol* 2000;13:107–112.
15. Attanoos RL, Gallateau-Salle F, Gibbs AR, et al. Primary thymic epithelial tumours of the pleura mimicking malignant mesothelioma. *Histopathology* 2002;41:42–49.
16. Mayall FG, Goddard H, Gibbs AR. Intermediate filament expression in mesothelioma: leiomyoid mesotheliomas are not uncommon. *Histopathology* 1992;21:453.
17. Ordonez NG. Immunohistochemical diagnosis of epithelioid mesotheliomas: a critical review of old markers, new markers. *Hum Pathol* 2002;33:953–967.
18. Rucko LP, De Laatp A, Matteucci C. Expression of Icam-1 and Vcam-1 in human malignant mesothelioma. *J Pathol* 1996;179:266–271.
19. Collins CL, Ordonez NG, Schaefer R, et al. Thrombomodulin expression in malignant pleural mesothelioma and pulmonary adenocarcinoma. *Am J Pathol* 1992;141:827–833.
20. Brown RW, Clarke GM, Tandon AK, et al. Multiple marker immunohistochemical phenotypes distinguishing malignant pleural mesothelioma from pulmonary adenocarcinoma. *Hum Pathol* 1993;24:347–354.
21. Ascoli V, Scalzo CC, Taccougna S, et al. The diagnostic value of thrombomodulin immunolocalisation in serous effusions. *Arch Pathol Lab Med* 1995;119:1136–1140.
22. Attanoos RL, Webb R, Dojcinov SD, et al. Malignant epithelioid mesothelioma: anti-mesothelial marker expression correlates with histological pattern. *Histopathology* 2001;39:584–588.
23. Attanoos RL, Webb R, Dojcinov SD, et al. Value of mesothelial and epithelial antibodies in distinguishing diffuse peritoneal mesothelioma in females from serous papillary carcinoma of the ovary and peritoneum. *Histopathology* 2002;40:237–244.
24. Attanoos RL, Goddard H, Gibbs AR. Mesothelioma binding antibodies: thrombomodulin OV632 and HBME1 and their use in the diagnosis of mesothelioma. *Histopathology* 1996;29: 209–215.
25. Chang K, Pai LH, Pass H. Monoclonal antibody K1 reacts with epithelial mesothelioma but not with lung adenocarcinoma. *Am J Surg Pathol* 1992;16:259–268.
26. Ordonez NG. Value of mesothelin immunostaining in the diagnosis of mesothelioma. *Mod Pathol* 2003;16:192–197.
27. Doglioni C, Dei Toss AP, Laurino L, et al. Calretinin: a novel immunocytochemical marker for mesothelioma. *Am J Surg Pathol* 1996;20:1037–1046.
28. Ordonez NG. Value of calretinin immunostaining in differentiating epithelial mesothelioma from lung adenocarcinoma. *Mod Pathol* 1998;11:929–933.
29. Barberis MC, Faleri M, Veronesi S, et al. Calretinin. A selective marker of normal and neoplastic mesothelial cells in serous effusions. *Acta Cytol* 1997;41:1757–1761.
30. Brockstedt U, Guluas M, Dobra K, et al. An optimised battery of 8 antibodies that can distinguish most cases of epithelial mesothelioma from adenocarcinoma. *Am J Clin Pathol* 2000;114:203–209.
31. Carella R, Deleonardi G, D'Rrico A, et al. Immunohistochemical panels for differentiating epithelial malignant mesothelioma from lung adenocarcinoma. A study with logistic regression analysis. *Am J Surg Pathol* 2000;25:43–50.
32. Miettenen M, Sarlomo-Rikala M. Expression of calretinin, thrombomodulin, keratin 5 and mesothelin lung carcinomas of different types: an immunohistochemical analysis of 596 tumours in comparison with epithelioid mesotheliomas of the pleura. *Am J Surg Pathol* 2003;27:150–158.
33. Kimura A. Podoplanin as a marker for mesothelioma. *Pathol Int* 2005;55:83–86.
34. Ordonez NG. The diagnostic utility of immunohistochemistry in distinguishing between epithelioid mesotheliomas and squamous carcinomas of the lung: a comparative study. *Mod Pathol* 2006;19:417–428.
35. Chu A Y, Litzky LA, Pasha TL, et al. Utility of D2-40, a novel mesothelial marker, in the diagnosis of malignant mesothelioma. *Mod Pathol* 2005;18:105–110.

36. Ordonez NG. D2-40 and podoplanin are highly specific and sensitive immunohistochemical markers of epithelioid malignant mesothelioma. *Hum Pathol* 2005;36:372–380.
37. Amin KM, Litzky LA, Smythe WR, et al. Wilm's tumour 1 susceptibility (WT1) gene products are selectively expressed in malignant mesothelioma. *Am J Pathol* 1995;14:6 344–356.
38. Foster MR, Johnson JE, Olson SJ, et al. Immunohistochemical analysis of nuclear v's cytoplasmic staining in WT1 in malignant mesotheliomas and primary pulmonary adenocarcinomas. *Arch Pathol Lab Med* 2001;125:1316–1320.
39. Ordonez NG. Value of thyroid transcription factor 1, e-cadherin, BG8, WT1 and CD44s immunostaining in distinguishing epithelial pleural mesothelioma from pulmonary and non pulmonary adenocarcinoma. *Am J Surg Pathol* 2000;24:598–606.
40. Ho CC, Kuo SH, Huang PH, et al. Caveolin-1 expression is significantly associated with drug resistance and poor prognosis in advanced non-small cell lung cancer patients treated with Gem cytogene based chemotherapy. *Lung Cancer* 2008;59:105–110.
41. Amatya VJ, Takeshima Y. Caveolin-1 is a novel immunohistochemical marker to differentiated epithelioid mesothelioma from lung adenocarcinoma. *Histopathology* 2009;55:10–19.
42. Bishop JA, Sharma R, Illei PB. Napsin A and thyroid transcription factor-1 expression in carcinomas of the lung, breast, pancreas, colon, kidney, thyroid and malignant mesothelioma. *Hum Pathol* 2010;41:20–25.
43. Yang M, Nonaka D. A study of immunohistochemical differential expression in pulmonary and mammary carcinomas. *Mod Pathol* 2010;23:654–661.
44. Yuan y, Nymoen DA, Staynes HT, et al. Tenascin X is a novel diagnostic marker of malignant mesothelioma. *Am J Surg Pathol* 2009;33:1673–1682.
45. Pass HI, Lott D, Lonardo F, et al. Asbestos exposure, pleural mesothelioma and serum osteopontin levels. *N Engl J Med* 2005;353:1564–1573.
46. Laury AR, Homick JL, Perets R, et al. PAX 8 reliably distinguishes ovarian serous tumours from malignant mesothelioma. *Am J Surg Pathol* 2010;34:627–635.
47. Yaziji H, Battifora H, Barry TS, et al. Evaluation of 12 antibodies for distinguishing epithelioid mesothelioma from adenocarcinoma: identification of a 3 antibody immunohistochemical panel with maximal sensitivity and specificity. *Mod Pathol* 2006;19:514–523.
48. Marchevsky AM, Wick MR. Evidence based guidelines for the utilisation of immunostains in diagnostic pathology: pulmonary adenocarcinoma vs mesothelioma. *Appl Immunohistochem Mol Morphol* 2007;15:140–144.
49. Klebe S, Nurminen M, Leigh J, et al. Diagnosis of epithelial mesothelioma using tree based regression analysis and a minimal panel of antibodies. *Pathology* 2009;41:140–148.
50. Klebe S, Brownlee NA, Mahar A, et al. Sarcomatoid mesothelioma: a clinical-pathologic correlation of 326 cases. *Mod Pathol* 2010;23:470–479.
51. Saad RS, Cho P, Liu YL, et al. The value of epithelial membrane antigen in separating benign mesothelial proliferation from malignant mesothelioma: a comparative study. *Diagn Cytopathol* 2005;32:156–159.
52. Attanoos RL, Griffin A, Gibbs AR. The use of immunohistochemistry in distinguishing reactive from neoplastic mesothelium. A novel use for desmin and comparative evaluation with epithelial membrane antigen, P53, platelet-derived growth factor receptor, P-glycoprotein and Bcl-2. *Histopathology* 2003;43:231–238.
53. Davidson B, Nielsen SCT, Christensen JCT, et al. The role of desmin and N-cadherin in effusion cytology: a comparative study using established markers of mesothelial and epithelial cells. *Am J Surg Pathol* 2001;25:1405–1412.
54. Kupryjaczyka J. Desmin expression in reactive mesothelium: a potential aid in evaluation of gynecologic specimens. *Int J Gynecol Path* 1998;17:123–128.
55. Kato Y, Tsuta K, Seki K, et al. Immunohistochemical detection of Glut 1 can discriminate between reactive mesothelium and malignant mesothelioma. *Mod Pathol* 2007;20:215–220.
56. Kumaki F, Kawai T Churg A, et al. Expression of Telomerase reverse transcriptase (TERT) in malignant mesothelioma. *Am J Surg Pathol* 2002;26:365–370.

Atypical Mesothelial Proliferations

13

Timothy Craig Allen

When appropriate histologic and immunohistochemical studies of a pleural proliferation have excluded the diagnosis of metastatic disease to the pleura, and the proliferation has been shown to be of mesothelial origin, it then must be determined whether the pleural proliferation is a malignant one, that is, diffuse malignant mesothelioma, or a benign, reactive one. In many cases of simple mesothelial cell hyperplasia and fibrous pleuritis, the diagnosis is straightforward. In some cases, however, the epithelioid or spindle cell pleural proliferation may be more diagnostically challenging. These atypical mesothelial proliferations are diagnostically important because they mimic pleural diffuse malignant mesothelioma.

Benign reactive epithelioid atypical mesothelial hyperplasia of the pleura mimics epithelioid diffuse malignant mesothelioma; and benign reactive spindle cell proliferations, as part of fibrous pleuritis, mimic sarcomatoid diffuse malignant mesothelioma. Given the dismal prognosis and attendant medicolegal consequences of the diagnosis of diffuse malignant mesothelioma, distinguishing atypical mesothelial proliferations from epithelioid diffuse malignant mesothelioma and fibrous pleuritis from sarcomatoid diffuse malignant mesothelioma is extremely important.[1,2] That diffuse malignant mesotheliomas often occur in association with reactive epithelioid atypical mesothelial cell proliferations and/or fibrous pleuritis complicates rendering an accurate diagnosis even further. The diagnoses of atypical mesothelial hyperplasia, fibrous pleuritis, or diffuse malignant mesothelioma should be rendered only after a careful and extremely thorough gross and microscopic examination, and with appropriate attention to clinical and radiologic findings. In some cases of diffuse malignant mesothelioma, its diagnosis is relatively straightforward and the differential diagnosis of atypical mesothelial hyperplasia or fibrous pleuritis is not seriously entertained; however, in other, more difficult cases, the pathologist will find it necessary to differentiate between a benign, reactive atypical mesothelial hyperplasia, fibrous pleuritis, and a malignant diffuse malignant mesothelioma. Differentiating between these entities can be extremely difficult; indeed, it can be one of the most difficult diagnostic challenges in pathology.[3,4]

There are a few other points the pathologist must consider when differentiating between diffuse malignant mesothelioma and atypical mesothelial hyperplasia/fibrous pleuritis. First, a history of asbestos exposure is not relevant, and neither a history of asbestos exposure nor a history without asbestos exposure should influence the pathologist's diagnosis. Second, with AMP, the terms "atypical mesothelial proliferation" and "atypical mesothelial hyperplasia" denote the same process, and the pathologist should not be confused in situations where the terms are used interchangeably. Third, mesothelioma in situ—markedly atypical mesothelial cells arranged in a single row along the pleural surface[4]—may in some cases be identified adjacent to obvious diffuse malignant mesothelioma; however, as its histologic features

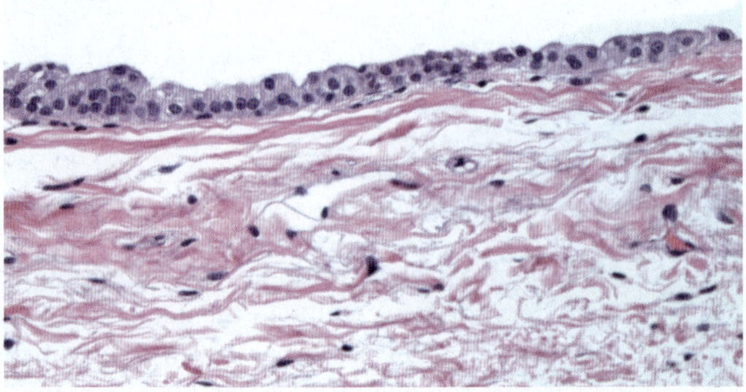

FIGURE 13-1: High-power image of so-called mesothelioma in situ. The area is adjacent to an area of invasive diffuse malignant mesothelioma, not shown in this figure. Compare with simple mesothelial hyperplasia (Fig. 13-7).

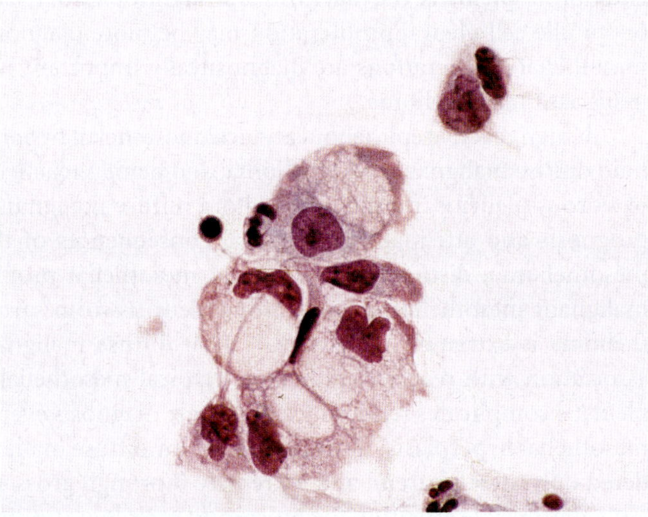

FIGURE 13-2: Markedly atypical reactive mesothelial cells in pleural fluid.

significantly overlap with those found with simple mesothelial hyperplasia and atypical mesothelial hyperplasia, the diagnosis of mesothelioma in situ should not be rendered (Fig. 13-1). Instead, biopsies containing only the histologic features of "mesothelioma in situ" should be diagnosed as atypical mesothelial hyperplasia. Fourth, as many of these patients have pleural effusions, and cytologic specimens are frequently submitted to the pathologist for diagnosis, it is extremely important to remember that, with possibly an exceedingly rare exception in the case of diffuse malignant mesothelioma, the diagnoses of diffuse malignant mesothelioma and atypical mesothelial hyperplasia/fibrous pleuritis cannot be made cytologically. The pathologist must also remember that benign mesothelial proliferations, both simple hyperplasia and atypical mesothelial hyperplasia, often show marked cytologic atypia, and conversely, diffuse malignant mesothelioma can exhibit particularly bland cytologic features (Figs. 13-2 and 13-3). Fifth, critical to proper diagnosis is adequate biopsy tissue. Needle biopsies are almost always too limited to be suitable for adequate diagnosis. Larger thoracoscopic biopsies are generally necessary for accurate diagnosis, and in some cases even

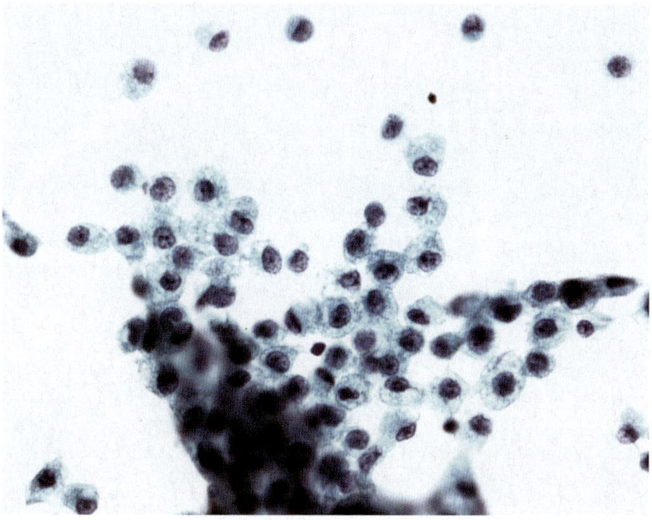

FIGURE 13-3: Relatively bland neoplastic diffuse malignant mesothelioma cells in pleural fluid.

these biopsies may be predominantly superficial and contain insufficient tissue for adequate histologic evaluation. Sixth, because benign reactive pleural conditions often cause pleural effusion and pleural thickening, mimicking diffuse malignant mesothelioma, in cases where significant pleural thickening is radiologically absent, the pathologist should be extremely cautious in diagnosing diffuse malignant mesothelioma. Early diffuse malignant mesotheliomas—which have not yet developed significant pleural thickening—do rarely occur; however, these cases are very rare. Finally, with difficult cases, referral of the case to a pulmonary pathologist with expertise in the diagnosis of diffuse malignant mesothelioma and atypical mesothelial hyperplasia is warranted. The United States–Canadian Mesothelioma Reference Panel and the International Mesothelioma Panel may be able to assist in diagnosing difficult cases. It is important to remember that where any doubt remains in the diagnosis of diffuse malignant mesothelioma, such a diagnosis should not be rendered, and instead the diagnosis of atypical mesothelial hyperplasia should be made. With the diagnosis of atypical mesothelial hyperplasia, the clinician can reassess the patient, and more tissue can then be obtained if necessary.

GROSS AND HISTOLOGIC FEATURES OF ATYPICAL MESOTHELIAL PROLIFERATIONS

As gross features of atypical mesothelial hyperplasia/fibrous pleuritis and diffuse malignant mesothelioma may overlap, gross examination is of limited usefulness in distinguishing these entities. Both diffuse malignant mesothelioma and atypical mesothelial hyperplasia/fibrous pleuritis frequently cause pleural effusions. However, pleural diffuse malignant mesothelioma typically shows significant pleural thickening that surrounds the lung in a rind-like pattern, a gross feature that may or may not be present with atypical mesothelial hyperplasia. As this feature may not be appreciable on limited biopsy tissue, clinical and radiologic correlation is very important (Figs. 13-4 to 13-6).

The primary tool in differentiating atypical mesothelial hyperplasia/fibrous pleuritis and diffuse malignant mesothelioma is histology. Unlike differentiating pleural diffuse malignant mesothelioma from the more common metastatic neoplasms to the pleura, where

FIGURE 13-4: Gross image of normal pleura, showing a thin membranous covering of the lung parenchyma.

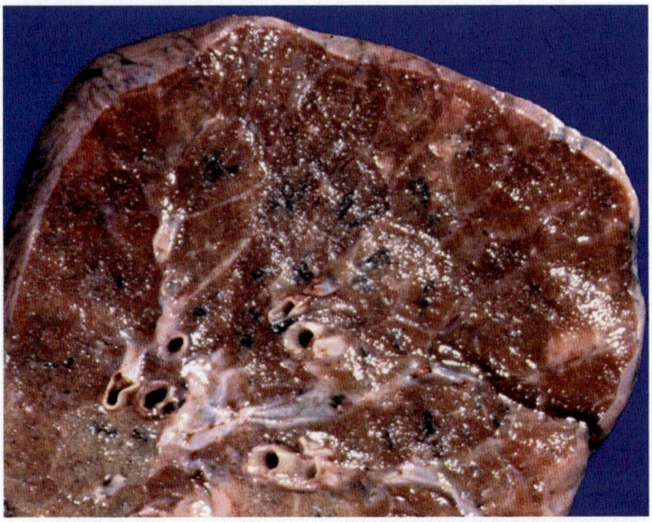

FIGURE 13-5: Gross image of fibrous pleuritis, showing ragged, irregular pleural surface made up of fibrous and fibrinous material.

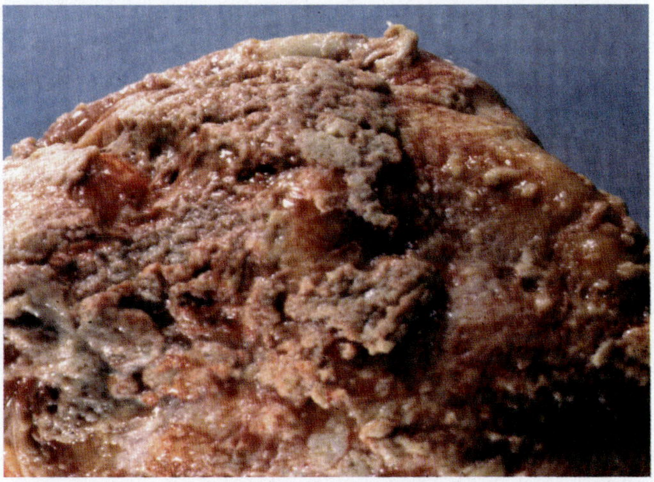

FIGURE 13-6: Gross image of diffuse malignant mesothelioma, showing rind-like thickening of pleura.

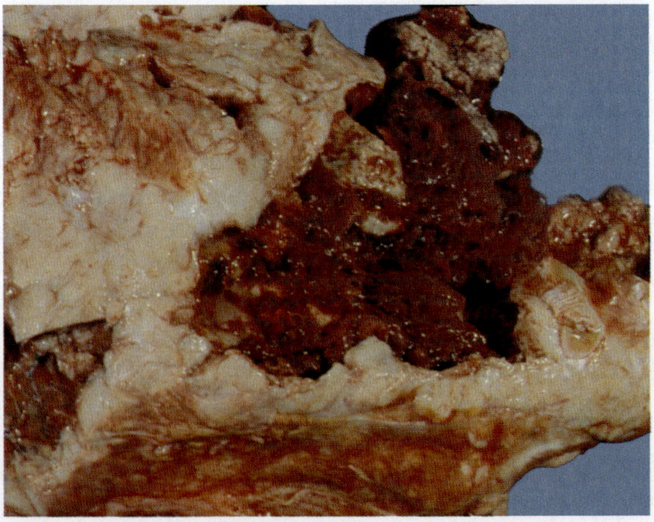

immunostains have come to play a vital role, differentiating atypical mesothelial hyperplasia/fibrous pleuritis from diffuse malignant mesothelioma incorporates a much more limited use of immunostaining. Benign reactive pleural lesions generally show varying combinations of reactive mesothelial cell hyperplasia and organizing pleuritis; however, in many cases, one or the other predominates. As their histologic features differ, the histology of epithelioid atypical mesothelial hyperplasias and pleural spindle cell proliferations, and their differentiation from epithelioid and sarcomatoid diffuse malignant mesothelioma, respectively, will be discussed individually.

ATYPICAL MESOTHELIAL PROLIFERATIONS

Any cause of irritation or injury to the pleura, including infections, pneumothorax, post-surgical injury, drug reaction, and collagen vascular diseases, may cause mesothelial cells to proliferate along the pleural surface. In cases where the mesothelial proliferation is limited to the pleural surface, and the mesothelial proliferation consists of generally uniform cuboidal to rounded cells, the diagnosis of simple mesothelial hyperplasia is appropriate (Fig. 13-7).

In many cases of pleural injury or irritation, however, there are variable amounts of fibrin deposition, granulation tissue, and pleural fibrosis, within which entrapped reactive mesothelial cells are frequently identified. Entrapped mesothelial cells may range from bland proliferations to markedly atypical proliferations of cells mimicking neoplastic cells, including diffuse malignant mesothelioma. These more atypical proliferations of mesothelial cells, for which malignancy is in the differential diagnosis, are termed atypical mesothelial hyperplasia. There are several histologic features important in the differentiation of atypical mesothelial hyperplasia from diffuse malignant mesothelioma. Histologic features suggesting benignity include absence of invasion into lung parenchyma or chest wall soft tissue, lack of desmoplastic response, inconspicuous mitotic figures, mild cytologic atypia, cellularity oriented toward the surface of the pleura, and pseudoinvasion characterized by entrapment of mesothelial cells within granulation tissue or fibrinous material and generally restricted to the planes or infoldings of tissue (Figs. 13-8 to 13-11). Histologic features suggesting malignancy include obvious invasion into lung parenchyma and chest wall soft tissue,

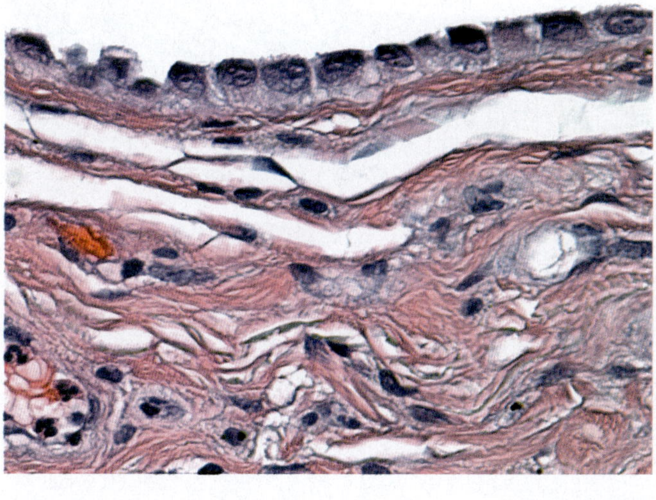

FIGURE 13-7: High-power image of simple mesothelial hyperplasia, showing an increased number of mesothelial cells, arranged in a single layer, with minimal atypia.

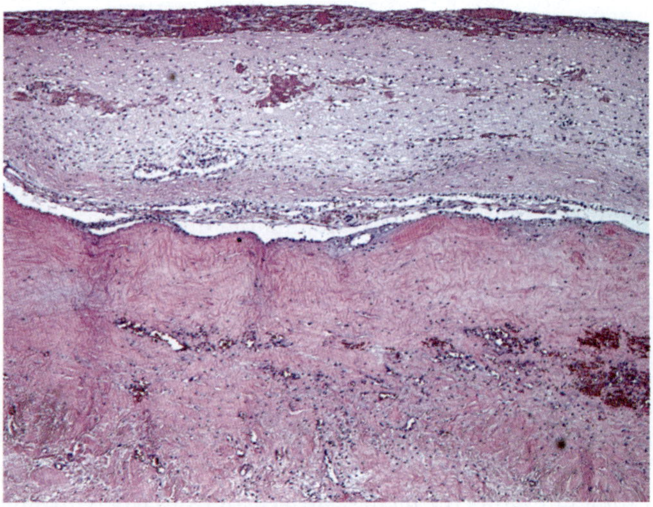

FIGURE 13-8: Medium-power image of atypical mesothelial hyperplasia, showing flattened groups of mesothelial cells that are oriented toward the pleural surface.

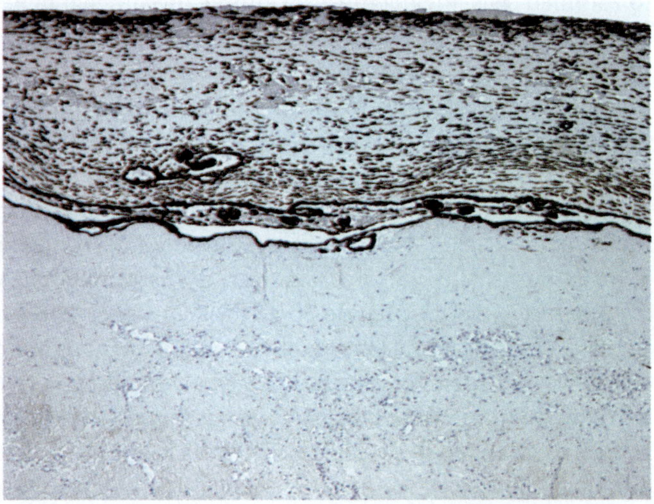

FIGURE 13-9: The same area as Figure 13-8, stained with cytokeratin, highlights the orientation of the mesothelial cells toward the surface and confirms the absence of mesothelial cell invasion.

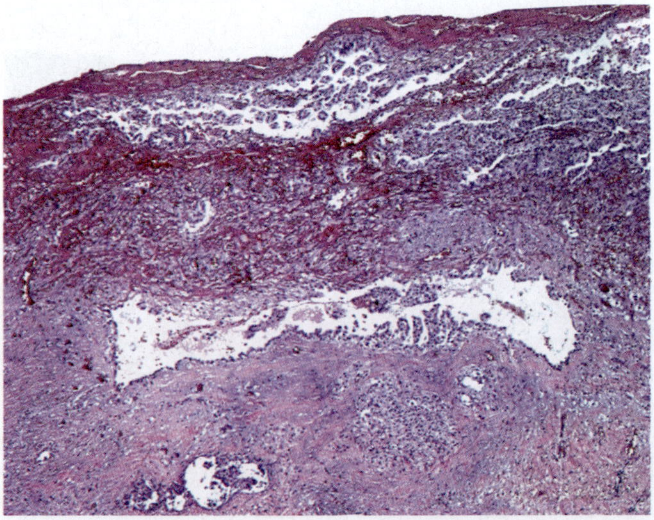

FIGURE 13-10: Medium power of pleura showing areas of mesothelial cell entrapment, which may mimic diffuse malignant mesothelioma.

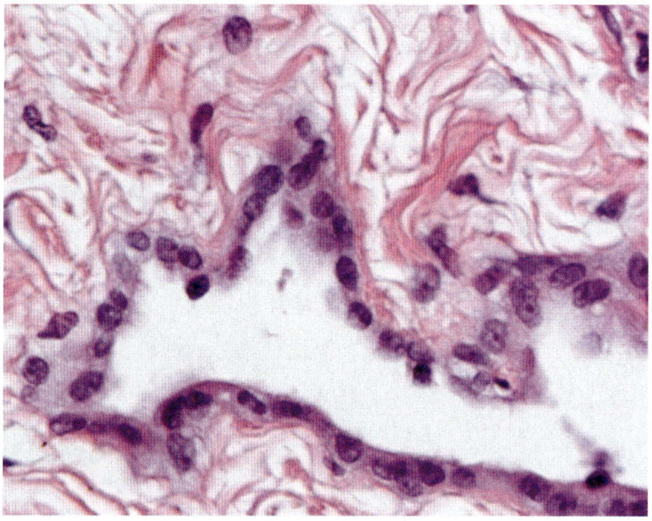

FIGURE 13-11: High-power image of entrapped mesothelial cells shows mild cytologic atypia and no mitotic figures.

desmoplasia, increased and abnormal mitotic figures, marked cytologic atypia or frankly malignant cytologic features, cellularity throughout the pleura without obvious orientation toward the pleural surface, and bland necrosis[1] (Table 13-1).

Once immunostains support a mesothelial origin of the atypical cells, immunostaining is of little benefit in differentiating epithelial atypical mesothelial hyperplasia from diffuse malignant mesothelioma. Keratin stain may assist in highlighting invasive diffuse malignant mesothelioma cells (Fig. 13-12). It is important to remember that these markedly reactive histologic features related to pleural injury do not exclude the presence of associated malignancy, including metastatic neoplasms and primary pleural neoplasms.

Table 13-1 Histologic features helpful in differentiating atypical mesothelial hyperplasia and epithelioid diffuse malignant mesothelioma

Histologic features
Features suggestive of benignity (atypical mesothelial hyperplasia):
Absence of invasion into lung parenchyma or chest wall soft tissue
Lack of desmoplastic response
Inconspicuous mitotic figures
Mild cytologic atypia
Cellularity oriented toward the surface of the pleura
Pseudoinvasion characterized by entrapment of mesothelial cells within granulation tissue or fibrinous material and generally restricted to the planes or infoldings of tissue
Features suggestive of malignancy (epithelioid diffuse malignant mesothelioma):
Obvious invasion into lung parenchyma and chest wall soft tissue
Desmoplasia
Increased and abnormal mitotic figures
Marked cytologic atypia or frankly malignant cytologic features
Cellularity throughout the pleura without obvious orientation toward the pleural surface
Bland necrosis

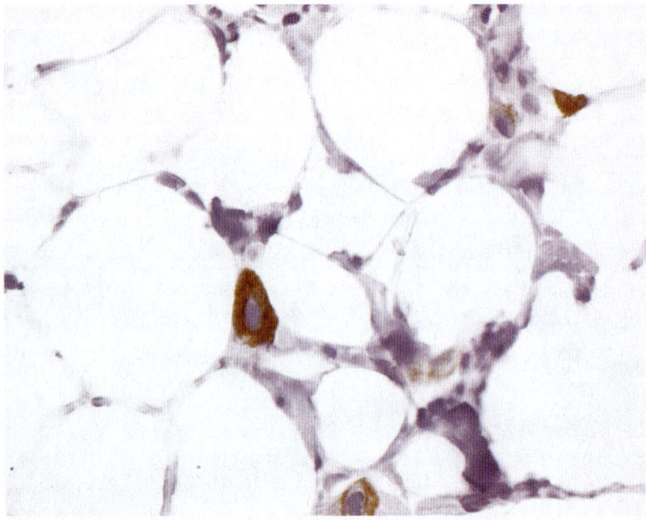

FIGURE 13-12: Immunostain with cytokeratin highlights diffuse malignant mesothelioma cells invading chest wall adipose tissue.

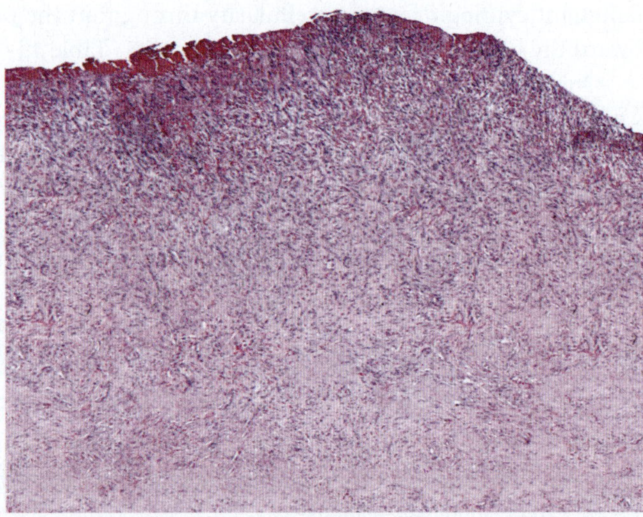

FIGURE 13-13: Low-power image of fibrous pleuritis showing decreasing cellularity away from the pleural surface. Compare with sarcomatoid diffuse malignant mesothelioma (Fig. 13-14).

FIBROUS PLEURITIS

Benign reactive sarcomatoid proliferations composed predominantly of spindle cells are generally fibrous pleuritis. However, sarcomatoid diffuse malignant mesothelioma, particularly desmoplastic diffuse malignant mesothelioma, may be extremely difficult to differentiate from fibrous pleuritis.[5] Both sarcomatoid diffuse malignant mesothelioma and fibrous pleuritis generally have relatively decreased cellularity and abundant collagen. Cellular orientation is important—fibrous pleuritis typically shows increased cellularity toward the pleural surface, with decreased cellularity toward the chest wall, whereas sarcomatoid diffuse malignant mesothelioma typically shows uniform cellularity throughout its thickness[5] (Figs. 13-13 and 13-14). Histologic features suggesting sarcomatoid or desmoplastic diffuse malignant mesothelioma include disorganized, invasive growth pattern; frankly sarcomatoid

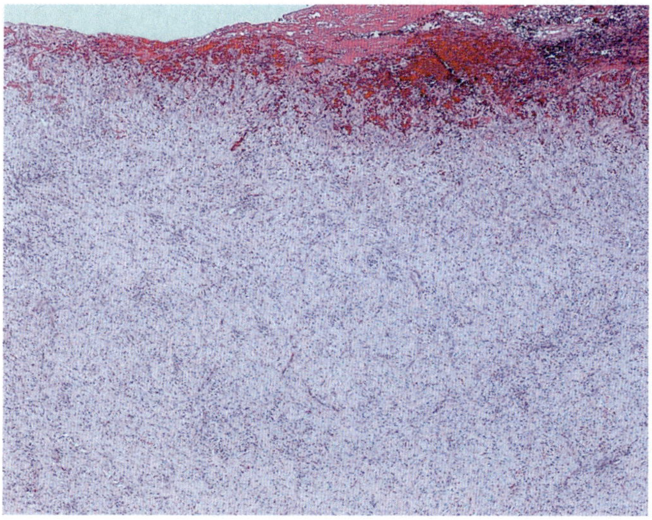

FIGURE 13-14: Low-power image of sarcomatoid diffuse malignant mesothelioma showing generally uniform cellularity throughout the thickened pleura. Compare with fibrous pleuritis (Fig. 13-13).

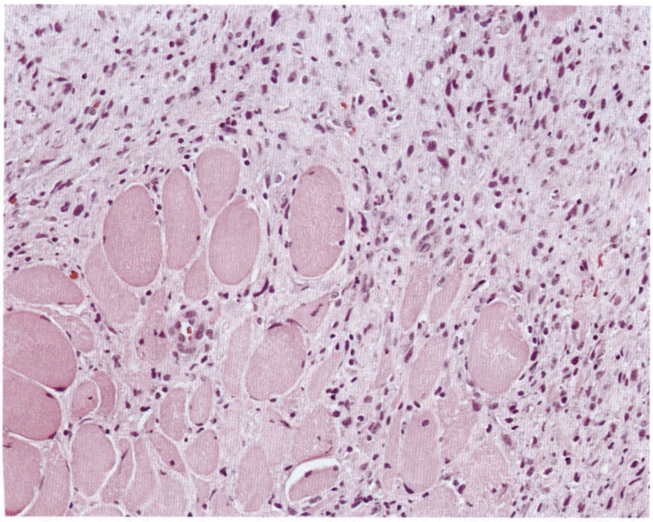

FIGURE 13-15: High-power image of sarcomatoid diffuse malignant mesothelioma, showing invasion of chest wall skeletal muscle.

areas, including marked nuclear atypia and atypical mitotic figures; and bland necrosis[5] (Figs. 13-15 to 13-17). Although metastatic disease is also considered a feature of sarcomatoid diffuse malignant mesothelioma, for the purposes of an original diagnosis on pleural biopsy, it is typically not a relevant diagnostic feature. Histologic features suggestive of benignity include uniform growth pattern with lack of invasion; mild cytologic atypia, with increased maturation in deeper cells; orientation of cellularity toward the pleural surface; inflammatory necrosis; and increased numbers of capillaries, with alignment perpendicular to the surface of the pleura[5] (Fig. 13-18; Table 13-2). Sarcomatoid diffuse malignant mesotheliomas are typically keratin immunopositive, and keratin immunostains can be quite valuable in helping the pathologist recognize invasive malignant cells within chest wall soft tissue and muscle, and lung parenchyma. These invasive tumor cells can be very bland cells

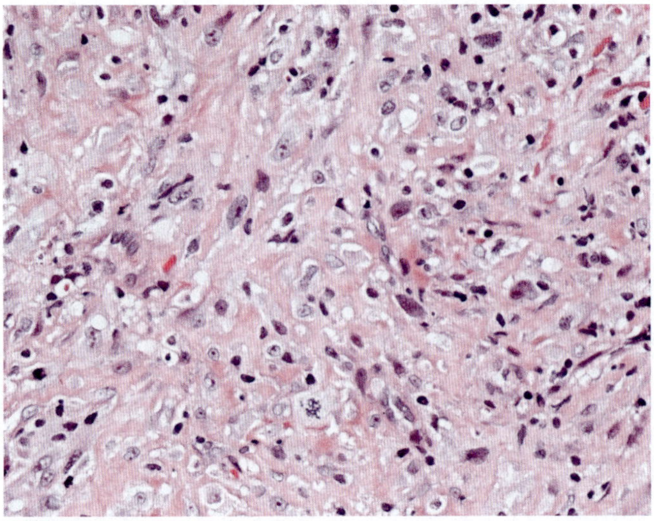

FIGURE 13-16: High-power image of sarcomatoid diffuse malignant mesothelioma, showing nuclear atypia and an atypical mitotic figure.

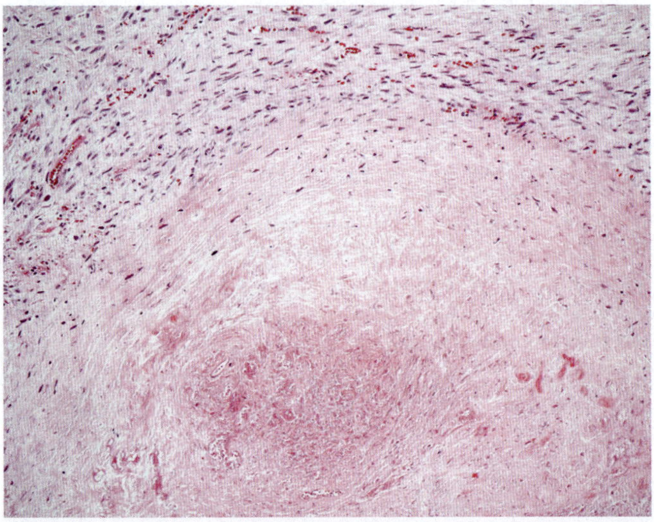

FIGURE 13-17: Bland necrosis within a sarcomatoid diffuse malignant mesothelioma.

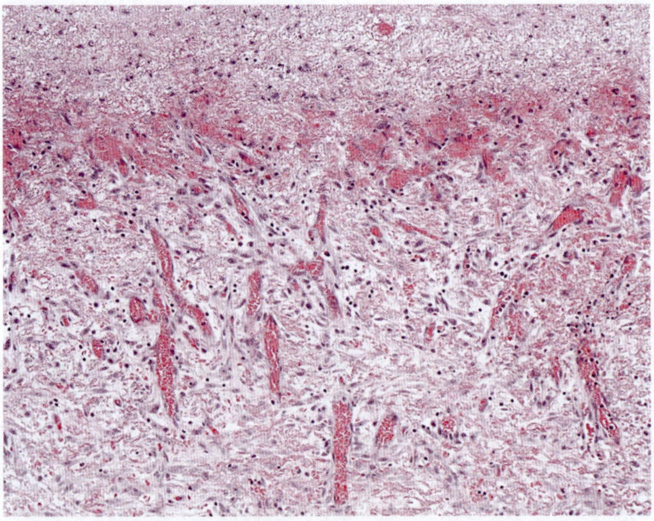

FIGURE 13-18: Blood vessels arranged perpendicularly to the pleural surface suggest the diagnosis of fibrous pleuritis rather than sarcomatoid diffuse malignant mesothelioma.

Table 13-2 Histologic features helpful in differentiating fibrous pleuritis and sarcomatoid diffuse malignant mesothelioma

Features suggestive of benignity (fibrous pleuritis): Uniform growth pattern, with lack of invasion into underlying lung parenchyma or chest wall Mild cytologic atypia, with increased maturation in deeper cells Orientation of cellularity toward the pleural surface Inflammatory necrosis Increased numbers of capillaries, with alignment perpendicular to the pleural surface
Features suggestive of malignancy (sarcomatoid diffuse malignant mesothelioma): Disorganized, invasive growth pattern Frankly sarcomatoid areas, with cytologic features including marked nuclear atypia and atypical mitotic figures Bland necrosis

and resemble fibroblasts. Tumor cells often insinuate themselves between chest wall adipocytes, with invasion of skeletal muscle fibers seen less often.[5] Sarcomatoid diffuse malignant mesothelioma tumor cells often invade the lung parenchyma by forming tumor cell nests within subpleural alveoli or bronchioles in a pattern resembling organizing pneumonia, or by tracking along secondary lobular septa.[5] Desmoplastic diffuse malignant mesotheliomas may also exhibit expansile nodules, which show an abrupt transition from areas of markedly increased cellularity to paucicellular, more desmoplastic, areas. Some cases of fibrous pleuritis may mimic sarcomatoid diffuse malignant mesothelioma closely, and extreme caution must be used to avoid overinterpretation of areas of fibrous pleuritis mimicking sarcomatoid diffuse malignant mesothelioma as true sarcomatoid diffuse malignant mesothelioma. If after careful examination any doubt remains, review by a pulmonary pathology expert is prudent (Figs. 13-19 to 13-24).

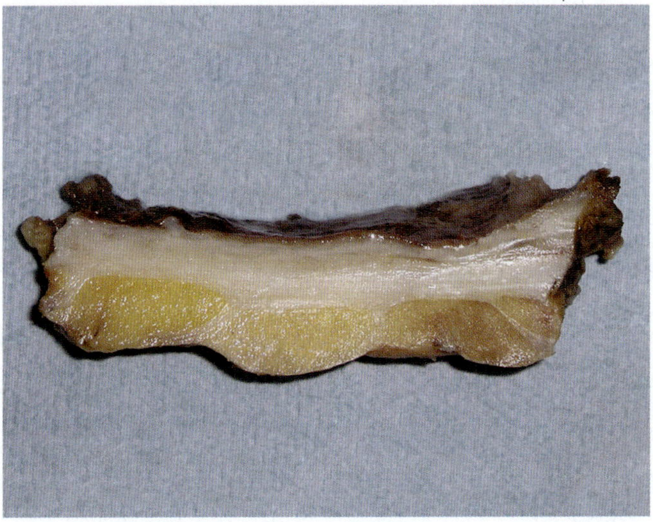

FIGURE 13-19: Gross image of a longstanding fibrous pleuritis, forming a pleural rind that mimics diffuse malignant mesothelioma.

FIGURE 13-20: Resolving fibrous pleuritis may contain areas with a "basket weave" pattern as well as cellular areas, mimicking sarcomatoid diffuse malignant mesothelioma.

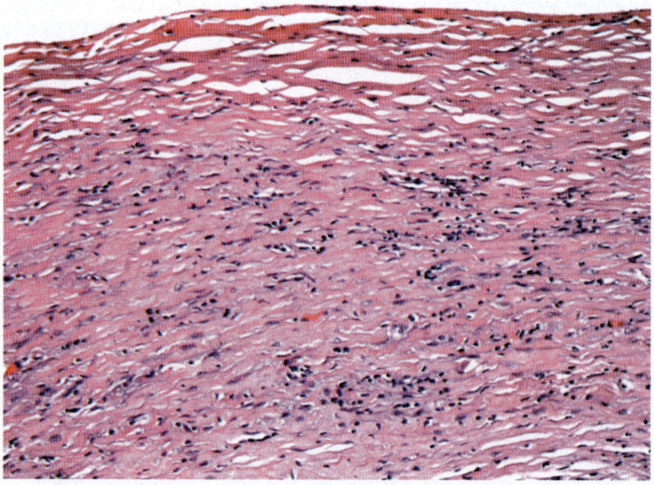

FIGURE 13-21: Entrapped mesothelial cells within fibrous pleuritis may form a complex pattern mimicking biphasic diffuse malignant mesothelioma.

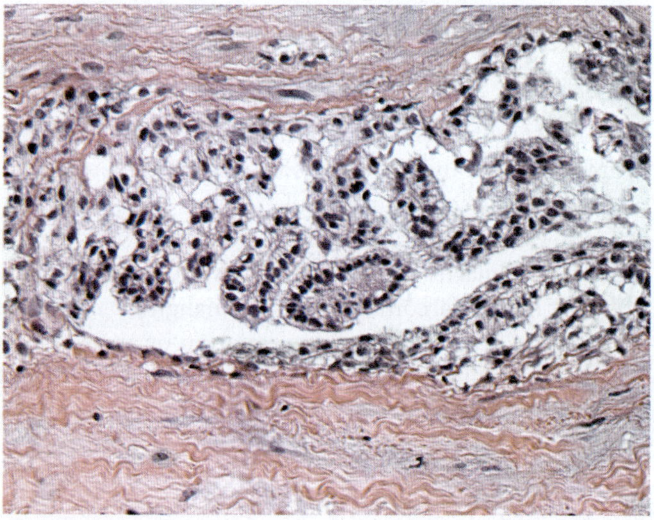

FIGURE 13-22: Fibrous pleuritis may involve adipose tissue, mimicking sarcomatoid diffuse malignant mesothelioma invading chest wall adipose tissue.

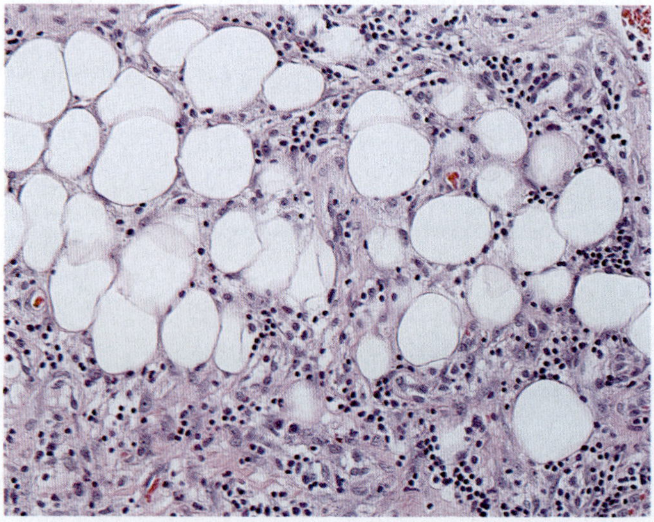

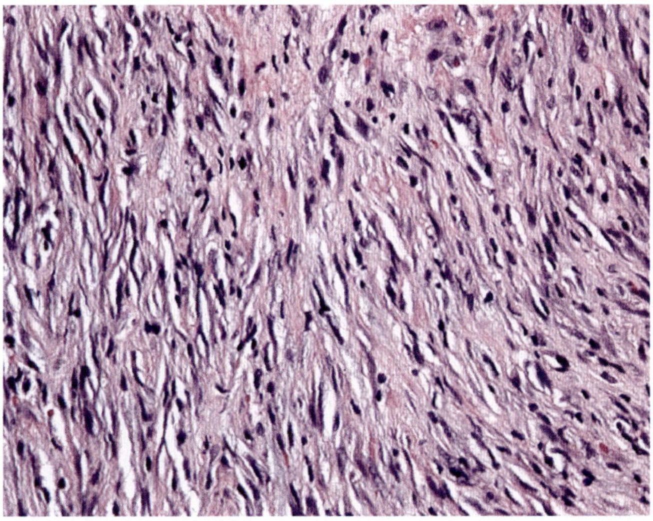

FIGURE 13-23: High power of an area of fibrous pleuritis with increased cellularity, mimicking sarcomatoid diffuse malignant mesothelioma.

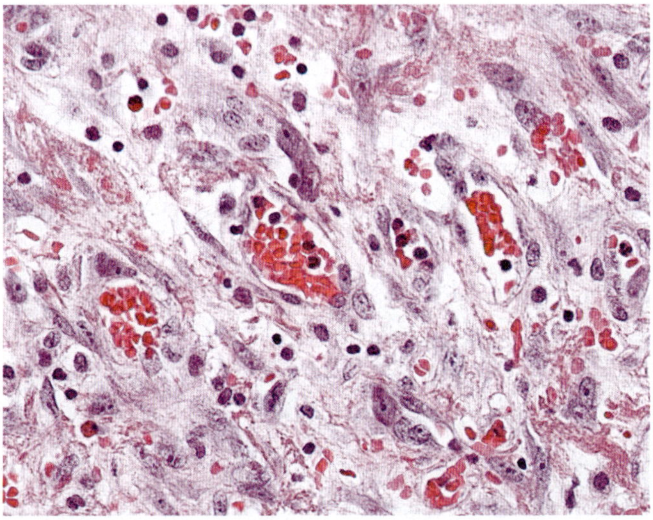

FIGURE 13-24: High power of fibrous pleuritis showing atypical cells that may mimic sarcomatoid diffuse malignant mesothelioma.

References

1. Cagle PT, Churg A. Differential diagnosis of benign and malignant mesothelial proliferations on pleural biopsies. *Arch Pathol Lab Med* 2005;129:1421–1427.
2. Separation of benign and malignant mesothelial proliferations. In: Churg A, Cagle PT, Roggli VL, eds. *Tumors of the Serosal Membranes.* Silver Spring, MD: ARP Press; 2006:83–101.
3. Kradin RL, Mark EJ. Distinguishing benign mesothelial hyperplasia from neoplasia: a practical approach. *Semin Diagn Pathol* 2006;23:4–14.
4. Henderson DW, Shilkin KB, Whitaker D. Reactive mesothelial hyperplasia vs mesothelioma, including mesothelioma in situ: a brief review. *Am J Clin Pathol* 1998;110:397–404.
5. Mangano WE, Cagle PT, Churg A, et al. The diagnosis of desmoplastic malignant mesothelioma and its distinction from fibrous pleurisy: a histologic and immunohistochemical analysis of 31 cases including p53 immunostaining. *Am J Clin Pathol* 1998;110:191–199.

SECTION

III

Molecular Features

Molecular Mechanisms of Pathogenesis

14

Alain C. Borczuk

The molecular pathogenesis of diffuse malignant mesothelioma is a multistep process that combines elements of inflammatory and cytokine-mediated tissue injury, loss of tumor suppressor gene activity, and eventual cellular dependency on a variety of growth factor pathways. These events have been examined in the context of understanding the origin and behavior of this tumor, and more recently, the specific pathways have been the subject of scrutiny as specific proteins may serve as prognostic markers and molecular therapeutic targets.

The chapter focuses on a stepwise progression toward the development of diffuse malignant mesothelioma. The complex interplay of molecular events is, in most cases, set into motion by asbestos exposure. In most cases, the development of diffuse malignant mesothelioma is linked to asbestos exposure, and much attention has been placed on the effect of fiber type, exposure level, and latency. These topics are important but to be covered in other chapters. In addition to asbestos, another fiber, erionite, is linked to diffuse malignant mesothelioma. The specifics of erionite exposure have led to insights regarding possible genetic susceptibility to diffuse malignant mesothelioma. Radiation exposure, largely in the therapeutic setting (after treatment for other malignancies), has also been linked to the development of diffuse malignant mesothelioma. Oncogenic effects of SV40 virus on mesothelioma cell lines have led to insights into pathways essential for diffuse malignant mesothelioma development, but its role as a cofactor in human disease remains controversial.

ASBESTOS-INDUCED MOLECULAR ALTERATIONS

The effect of asbestos exposure in causing cellular transformation is complex and supported by several lines of study. The observation that asbestos fiber exposure is toxic to mesothelial cells is a starting point that must be reconciled with the fact that this is an early event in tumor development. The effect of asbestos on mesothelial cells in culture is apoptotic cell death,[1] and this is mediated by the development of reactive oxygen species.[2] Once it is recognized that oncogenic events such as KRAS activation may increase sensitivity to apoptosis in normal cells[3] and that oncogenic C-myc or Wnt pathway activation can lead to cellular senescence,[4] it becomes clearer that cells must survive such events as part of malignant transformation. Cellular events in the correct context can lead to cell death, but survival (either inherent in a stem cell or acquired by local signals) can allow for progression from this initiating event in a prooncogenic/prosurvival milieu.

In the case of diffuse malignant mesothelioma, asbestos may have an effect on multiple cell types. There may be a direct effect of asbestos fibers on mesothelial cell mitosis by interfering with the mitotic spindle, resulting in abnormal cell division and aneuploidy.[5] However, more intriguing is the release of TNF-α by macrophages attempting to ingest fibers, as well as the concomitant induction of TNF-α and its receptor on mesothelial cells themselves. The effect of TNF-α via the NF-kB pathway is cellular survival. In normal cells, NF-kB is inactive due to cytoplasmic localization of its components bound with IkK proteins or as precursor proteins like p105. With the correct stimulus, phosphorylation of IkK and p105 leads to ubiquitination that leads to targeting for proteasomal degradation.[6] Without IkK proteins or after proteolytic cleavage of precursor proteins, components of NF-kB translocate to the nucleus where they serve as transcription factors. The activation of NF-kB transcriptional effect is generally antiapoptotic, promoting cell survival. The TNF-α–rich environment created initially by the macrophages, coupled with the induction of TNF receptor on the mesothelial cells themselves (a paracrine effect), allows for mesothelial cell survival[7]; the subsequent mesothelial production of TNF-α eventually makes this an autocrine activation.

The cytotoxic effect of asbestos is related to the generation of reactive oxygen species (at least in part through the ionic state of iron). Cells surviving reactive oxygen species (ROS) cytotoxicity through NFkB pathway leaves them exposed to effects of reactive oxygen species. Asbestos causes a dose-dependent increase in H_2O_2. Reactive oxygen species can cause DNA injury and have been shown to cause mutations in test systems.[8] More relevant to mesothelioma pathogenesis, both crocidolite asbestos and H_2O_2 have been shown to cause similar rates of mutation in these test systems, both of which are reversed by catalase, implicating ROS (H_2O_2) as a cause.[9] These mutations are characteristically G-T transversions.[10]

A third mechanism of asbestos-induced injury is related to increased ERK (extracellular signal–related kinase)-mediated phosphorylation of transcription factors that are part of the AP-1 complex. This complex can be formed by proteins encoded by c-jun and c-fos. The role of AP-1 in development of malignant cells is multifactorial and involves regulation of transcription of growth-related, apoptotic, and inflammatory pathways.[11] In the case of the development of mesothelioma, induction of AP-1 by TNF-α appears relevant in light of the TNF-α role in the microenvironment causing initiation of asbestos-induced injury, and the effect of AP-1 activation includes repression of p53 and its pathway and potential effects on the $p16^{INK4}$/Rb pathway as well. Specifically, Fra-1 (Fos-related antigen) phosphorylation has been implicated in mesothelial cell transformation.[12]

It has been previously noted that diffuse malignant mesothelioma is unusual in that the typical mutations that are seen in many other solid tumors (e.g., p53, Kras, and epidermal growth factor receptor [EGFR]) have not been detected in diffuse malignant mesothelioma.[13] However, it is clear that perturbations in these pathways do occur in diffuse malignant mesothelioma and that initial p53 and $p16^{INK4}$/Rb suppression may be a consequence of the cellular survival induced by asbestos exposure and the inflammatory microenvironment generated.

Having established a connection between DNA injury and asbestos exposure, the injury in diffuse malignant mesothelioma appears to more often deletion of tumor suppressor genes than acquisition of mutations in oncogenes. Several studies using different techniques including conventional comparative genomic hybridization (CGH) and array-based CGH have found consistent alterations in diffuse malignant mesothelioma that include a spectrum of gains and losses that are summarized in Table 14-1. In a study using array CGH, Taniguchi et al.[14] identified two areas of high-level gains in 1p32.1 and 11q.22. The area of 1p32.1 corresponds to the c-jun gene (mentioned as part of AP-1 complex), and 11q.22 includes IAP2 and IAP3 (inhibitor of apoptosis). The finding of gains in the region of IAP2 and IAP3 (two similar genes, which likely arose from duplication) is a critical observation in the pathogenesis of diffuse malignant mesothelioma (MM). Linking again to the hypothesis that asbestos-mediated induction of TNF-α and NF-kB pathway activation are critical to mesothelial cellular survival after asbestos

Table 14-1 Recurrent gains and losses in diffuse malignant mesothelioma[14,17,18]

		Possible Gene Affected
Gains	1p32	JUN
	1q23	
	5p15	
	7p14-15	
	7q21,7q31	MET
	8q22-24	MYC
	11q22	IAP
	15q22-25	
	20p	
Losses	1p21	
	1p36	KIT
	3p21	
	4q22	TMSL3
	4q34	
	6q25	PLEKHG1
	9p21.3	P16/p14
	10p13	
	13q13-14	
	14q	
	18q	
	22q	NF2

exposure, IAP2 serves to mediate NF-kB effects. Specifically, TNF-α induction of NF-kB is significantly reduced without IAP proteins, and the function of IAP is critical to the activation of NF-kB pathway–mediated cell survival.[15] The importance of increased IAP gene expression in MM has also been discovered through gene expression profiling of cell lines and tumors.[16]

Most notable among losses include regions in 3p21, 4q, 6q, 9p, 10p, 13q, 14q, and 22q. These regions contain tumor suppressor genes that have become particularly relevant in MM and include neurofibromatosis 2 (Nf2 gene, protein merlin), $p16^{INK4}$, $p14^{ARF}$, and p15.[14,17,18]

The frequent 22q loss in MM is linked to loss of the NF2 gene, and a truncation as well as mutation/in-frame deletion of merlin (NF2 protein) is seen in a high number of MM cell lines and tumors.[19,20] NF2 is a critical regulator of contact-dependent inhibition of proliferation with a role that links cellular adhesion, receptor-mediated signaling, and the actin cytoskeleton. Whether by deletion, mutation, or functional inactivation, loss of NF2 is an important part of mesothelioma pathogenesis. In cases in which NF2 is structurally conserved, functional inactivation may occur through phosphorylation, and this may be mediated by the oncogene CPI-17.[21] In addition, an interesting study using microRNA profiling suggested that miRNA expression in mesothelioma may play a role in the suppression of NF2 and $p16^{INK4}$ expression.[22]

FIGURE 14-1: P16 and P15 effect on Rb. In the left panel, p16 and p15 inactivate Cdk4/6. Without Rb phosphorylation, Rb binds E2F and keeps cells in G0/G1. With loss of p16 and p15, Cdk4/6 activity allows for Rb phosphorylation and release from E2F, allowing cell cycle progression.

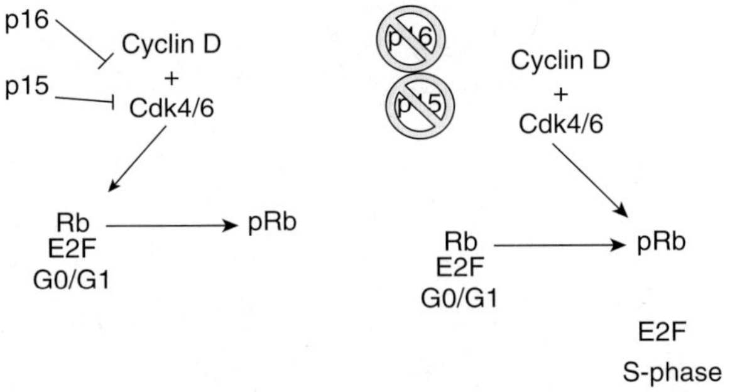

The frequent area of deletion in the area of chromosomal locus 9p21 encompasses three important tumor suppressor genes—p16^{INK4}, p15, and p14^{ARF}. While it is possible to preserve p15 function in the setting of p16^{INK4} loss, p14^{ARF} is an alternate reading frame that overlaps with p16^{INK4}, and therefore, deletion of p16^{INK4} is accompanied by loss of p14^{ARF}.[23]

The retinoblastoma (RB) gene is an important tumor suppressor gene whose function is to bind E2F transcription factors preventing progression of cell cycle (Fig. 14-1). The RB protein is phosphorylated by CDK4/6 and then by CDK2; phosphorylated RB eventually is prevented from binding and inactivating E2F and cell cycle progress. P16^{INK4} normally inhibits CDK4/6 and this inhibition prevents RB phosphorylation and therefore allows for continued blockade of E2F. p16^{INK4} loss results in loss of CDK4/6 inhibition, phosphorylation of RB, loss of E2F inhibition, and cell cycle progression.

There are several lines of evidence that p16^{INK4} loss is important in diffuse malignant mesothelioma. In 1995, Xio et al. demonstrated p16^{INK4} deletion in 72% of MM, with 100% of spindled/sarcomatoid MM with p16^{INK4} loss. Loss may be due to deletion in many cases, but promoter hypermethylation may be an important mechanism in other cases, resulting in loss of p16^{INK4} expression. Mutations do not appear to be common. Reexpression of p16^{INK4} in diffuse malignant mesothelioma cells results in cell death.[24] Animal models also support the importance of p16^{INK4} loss in the pathogenesis of diffuse malignant mesothelioma, as discussed more fully below.

Another interesting aspect of p16^{INK4} expression in diffuse malignant mesothelioma is the association with tumor progression/prognosis. In diffuse malignant mesothelioma–derived cell lines, p16^{INK4} loss is seen in virtually all cases, and this rate is higher than that seen in the actual tumors. While a criticism of gene expression profiling studies is inconsistency in gene lists and results, in this instance, gene expression profiling has found identical results in pleural and peritoneal diffuse malignant mesothelioma—that is, loss of p16^{INK4} expression is associated with poor survival independent of histologic subtype, with p16^{INK4} deletion in pleural disease and loss of immunoreactivity as a marker in peritoneal disease.[25–27] In addition, biphasic histology in peritoneal disease is almost always associated with p16^{INK4} loss.

p14^{ARF} has critical effects on the p53 pathway. As previously noted, p53 mutations are not common in diffuse malignant mesothelioma, but loss of this important pathway may be mediated via p14^{ARF} loss. One important normal function of p14^{ARF} is to bind MDM2. MDM2 normally degrades p53, and p14^{ARF} binding of MDM2 allows for maintenance of p53 protein level. P53 maintenance allows for p21 and Bax activation and resulting in control of cell growth and apoptosis. p14^{ARF} may also have direct apoptotic effects. p14^{ARF} reexpression causes increase in stable p53 and p21, with cell cycle control and apoptotic cell death in mesothelioma cell lines.[28]

By deletion of this one locus, p16^{INK4} loss results in RB inactivation and cell cycle progression, and p14^{ARF} loss results in degradation of p53 allowing for cell cycle progression and prevention of apoptosis. With deletion, loss of the tumor suppressor effect becomes relatively irreversible. In addition, loss of p15, a protein of similar function to p16^{INK4} and frequently codeleted with p16^{INK4}, may also contribute to the loss of tumor suppressor effect from this locus.

MOUSE MODELS

The critical role of merlin, p16^{INK4}, and p53 loss in the development of diffuse malignant mesothelioma is supported by animal models of diffuse malignant mesothelioma. Heterozygous mice for Nf2 (with only one functional Nf2 allele) exposed to asbestos develop MM with frequent loss of the wild-type Nf2 gene in the tumors. In addition, loss of Nf2 also occurs in asbestos-exposed wild-type mice. These tumors develop deletion of p16^{INK4}, p15, and p14^{ARF} (p19Arf in mice). A subset of tumors in these mice has retention of p14^{ARF} but loss of Tp53 function by another mechanism.[29]

Using a different method, Jongsma et al.[30] induced loss of Nf2, p53, and p16/p14 in a mouse model. Interestingly, Nf2 and p53 loss resulted in MM, and the additional loss of p16^{INK4} resulted in poorer survival and tumors with sarcomatoid histologic component.

SV40-INDUCED MOLECULAR CHANGES

Simian virus 40 (SV40) is a DNA virus classified as a polyoma virus. It has been extensively studied since, in certain animals, it can cause malignancy and, in cell lines, can cause cellular transformation. This is dependent on two critical virus-encoded proteins known as SV40 Large T antigen (Tag) and SV40 small t antigen (tag). These proteins have a role in suppressing p53 activity. Based on the discussion in the section of asbestos-induced pathogenesis, the ultimate suppression of p53 activity plays a key role in diffuse malignant mesothelioma pathogenesis, and mutation is not the path toward suppression in the majority of diffuse malignant mesotheliomas. While p14^{ARF} loss may play a role in p53 suppression, this may not be the only pathway (only about 70% have p16/p14 deletion), and p53 suppression may be mediated by other causes early in tumorigenesis even in tumors that ultimately develop a p14^{ARF} loss.

While this provides part of a theoretical basis for SV40 infection playing a causative role in human diffuse malignant mesothelioma, this area remains controversial. It is clear that SV40 infection in mesothelial cells in vitro can cause many of the pathway alterations critical to development of diffuse malignant mesothelioma and, at a minimum, has contributed a great deal to our understanding of diffuse malignant mesothelioma pathogenesis. SV40 tag can produce loss of p53 activity and importantly can also bind RB preventing its suppression of E2F transcription. SV40 tag can cause increase in AP-1 transcription factors as well.[31] This constellation of inhibitions and activations are central to diffuse malignant mesothelioma pathogenesis. Some groups have described detection of SV40 DNA and proteins from patient samples of diffuse malignant mesothelioma.[32]

The controversy in this area regards whether these in vitro observations are proof that this is causative of disease in humans in light of the human tumor observations that suggest false positives, which may have resulted from technical issues. It has been observed that SV40 can be detected in the blood of normal human populations[33] and that this rate is not higher in the blood and tumors of MM patients,[34] after allowances are made for technical problems in PCR detection. In 2004, Lopez Rios et al.[35] used primers for SV40-encoded genes that were not contained in commonly used laboratory plasmids, and the rate of SV40 detection in MM fell substantially, to about 6%. They failed to confirm detection of SV40-related proteins in diffuse malignant mesothelioma. Other groups have used similar techniques and determined that Large T antigen sequences were not present in diffuse malignant mesothelioma and in other tissues from mesothelioma-affected patients. Immunohistochemistry was negative with an SV40-specific antibody and that p53 activity was not suppressed in mesothelioma cell lines purported to contain SV40 previously.[36]

Based on these controversies, it is difficult to conclude at this time that SV40 infection plays a critical role in human diffuse malignant mesothelioma pathogenesis. It is, however, possible to state that SV40 can cause cellular transformation and does so in pathways that are likely to be relevant in human disease.

RADIATION

There is evidence that certain radiation exposures can increase the risk for diffuse malignant mesothelioma. In a recent review, data were examined from Thorotrast-exposed patients, atomic energy workers, and therapeutic radiation of cancer patients and subsequent risk of diffuse malignant mesothelioma. While this examination revealed some problems of methodology, the conclusion was that radiation-treated patients were at increased risk of diffuse malignant mesothelioma.[37] In another 2009 study, a 30-fold increased risk of diffuse malignant mesothelioma was reported after radiation for Hodgkin lymphoma, with a latency period of 10 to 34 years.[38] Differences in mutational or cytogenetic alteration between radiation-induced and asbestos-associated diffuse malignant mesothelioma have not been specifically examined, so differences in molecular pathogenesis cannot be commented on at this time.

GENETIC SUSCEPTIBILITY

One of the most intriguing developments in the pathogenesis of diffuse malignant mesothelioma lies in the examination of potential individual genetic susceptibility to diffuse malignant mesothelioma development. As chronicled by Dr. Carbone and colleagues, studies of erionite exposure and subsequent development of diffuse malignant mesothelioma in villages in Turkey have revealed possible genetic links to mesothelioma susceptibility. Erionite is a fibrous mineral that resembles glass-like fibers and has some properties similar to asbestos. This material was used in buildings in Turkish villages, and exposure to this mineral causes an increased risk of diffuse malignant mesothelioma. In fact, in animal studies, the risk of diffuse malignant mesothelioma is higher from erionite exposure than asbestos exposure. While familial clustering of diffuse malignant mesothelioma cases was originally linked to shared domiciles, several lines of evidence including exposure levels and careful familial cohort examination strongly suggest a genetic contribution.[39] Additional data derived from Tuzkoy, a large village in Turkey in which townspeople were erionite exposed, demonstrated an increased risk of diffuse malignant mesothelioma with HLA subtypes of HLAB41, HLAB58, and HLADR16 and decreased risk with subtypes B27, B35, and B44 when compared to nondiseased inhabitants and a database of Turkish renal donors.[40] Associations of diffuse malignant mesothelioma risk and levels of microsomal epoxide hydrolase and *N*-acetyltransferase 2 polymorphisms have led to conflicting results, with possible associations with XRCC1 and XRCC3 polymorphisms.[41]

GROWTH FACTORS

While examination of diffuse malignant mesothelioma pathogenesis focusing on initiation/risk factors for diffuse malignant mesothelioma and cytogenetic alterations resulting in tumor suppressor loss (resistance to apoptosis and loss of cell cycle control) may provide insight into potential preventative, diagnostic, prognostic, and therapeutic approaches to this disease, an examination of the growth factor milieu that results in continued growth support for this tumor is also critical toward developing rational approaches to treatment. While many growth factor pathways have been linked to diffuse malignant mesothelioma, there appears to a convergence of information regarding epidermal growth factor (EGF), insulin-like growth factor (IGF), hepatocyte growth factor (HGF), and vascular endothelial growth factor (VEGF).

EPIDERMAL GROWTH FACTOR

The EGFR is a cell surface protein that mediates signals from EGF and TGF-alpha, resulting in cellular proliferation. Overexpression of EGFR has been demonstrated in MM, especially the epithelioid type.[42,43] Also of interest is the finding that asbestos may induce EGFR expression in mesothelial cells.[44] However, while increased expression has been described in both peritoneal and pleural diffuse malignant mesothelioma, activating mutations have not been identified in pleural diffuse malignant mesothelioma.[45] In addition, treatment with erlotinib, a tyrosine kinase inhibitor targeting EGFR, has not been associated with response,[46] and treatment with gefitinib has only a modest effect on overall survival.[47] An interesting recent publication showed EGFR mutation in peritoneal diffuse malignant mesothelioma, with one classical L858R-activating mutation and seven novel mutations in the tyrosine kinase domain; this was associated with resectability, but no data on EGFR TKI response were published in that series.[48]

INSULIN-LIKE GROWTH FACTOR

Microarray studies have implicated the IGF pathway as important in diffuse malignant mesothelioma. Diffuse malignant mesotheliomas show increases in IGF-1 as well as IGFR. The combination of IGF secretion and expression of IGF receptor can result in autocrine growth effects on tumor cells as well as growth effects on adjacent stroma. Interestingly, IGF signals in cells with an increase in IRS-1 (insulin receptor substrate 1) are more growth related, while those with increased IRS 2 are more likely increase motility.[49]

HEPATOCYTE GROWTH FACTOR

HGF and its receptor Met are both increased in diffuse malignant mesothelioma suggesting the possibility of an autocrine loop. In addition, HGF mediates its effects via Fra-1, and Fra-1 phosphorylation (as an AP-1–related protein) has a role in diffuse malignant mesothelioma pathogenesis.[12] Given the possibility of pharmacologic targeting in this pathway, this may represent a therapeutic target in the future.

VASCULAR ENDOTHELIAL GROWTH FACTOR

VEGF promotes angiogenesis and, in the case of diffuse malignant mesothelioma, is produced by tumor. In addition, receptors for VEGF have also been identified on diffuse malignant mesothelioma tumor cells, suggesting possible autocrine effects.[50] VEGF is elevated in serum of mesothelioma patients as well as in effusions. TNF-alpha may increase IL6 production and IL-6 may induce VEGF production in diffuse malignant mesothelioma.[51] Whether an autocrine growth effect or angiogenic effect of VEGF, blockade of VEGF is a potential therapeutic approach under investigation.

SUMMARY

The pathogenesis of diffuse malignant mesothelioma, based on insights from in vitro studies, SV40 models, animal models, and studies of human tumors, is based on initiation events that confer survival and growth advantage in mesothelial cells that are followed by a series of losses in tumor suppressor genes NF2 and genes important for p53 function and RB pathway control. Tumor growth is maintained through diverse growth factor pathways, and these may serve as a road map guide toward effective targeted therapy (Fig. 14-2).

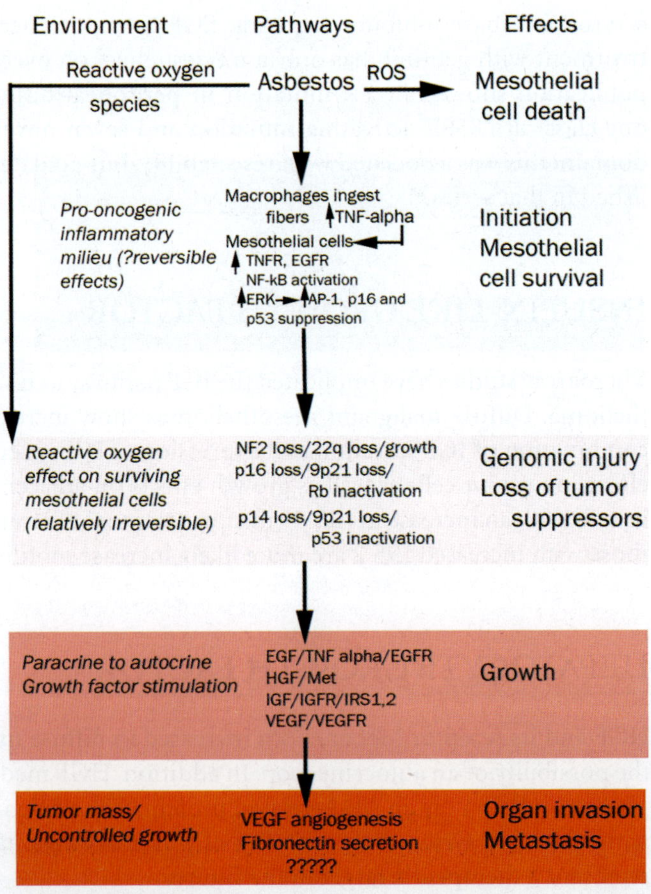

FIGURE 14-2: Summary of steps in asbestos-induced diffuse malignant mesothelioma pathogenesis.

References

1. BeruBe KA, Quinlan TR, Fung H, et al. Apoptosis is observed in mesothelial cells after exposure to crocidolite asbestos. *Am J Respir Cell Mol Biol* 1996;15:141–147.
2. Broaddus VC, Yang L, Scavo LM, et al. Asbestos induces apoptosis of human and rabbit pleural mesothelial cells via reactive oxygen species. *J Clin Invest* 1996;98:2050–2059.
3. Nesterov A, Nikrad M, Johnson T, et al. Oncogenic Ras sensitizes normal human cells to tumor necrosis factor-alpha-related apoptosis-inducing ligand-induced apoptosis. *Cancer Res* 2004;64: 3922–3927.
4. Campaner S, Doni M, Hydbring P, et al. Cdk2 suppresses cellular senescence induced by the c-myc oncogene. *Nat Cell Biol* 2010;12(Suppl):54–59; 1–14.
5. Ault JG, Cole RW, Jensen CG, et al. Behavior of crocidolite asbestos during mitosis in living vertebrate lung epithelial cells. *Cancer Res* 1995;55:792–798.
6. Scheidereit C. IkappaB kinase complexes: gateways to NF-kappaB activation and transcription. *Oncogene* 2006;25:6685–6705.
7. Yang H, Bocchetta M, Kroczynska B, et al. TNF-alpha inhibits asbestos-induced cytotoxicity via a NF-kappaB-dependent pathway, a possible mechanism for asbestos-induced oncogenesis. *Proc Natl Acad Sci U S A* 2006;103:10397–10402.
8. Kamp DW, Israbian VA, Preusen SE, et al. Asbestos causes DNA strand breaks in cultured pulmonary epithelial cells: role of iron-catalyzed free radicals. *Am J Physiol* 1995;268:L471–L480.
9. Xu A, Zhou H, Yu DZ, et al. Mechanisms of the genotoxicity of crocidolite asbestos in mammalian cells: implication from mutation patterns induced by reactive oxygen species. *Environ Health Perspect* 2002;110:1003–1008.
10. Unfried K, Schurkes C, Abel J. Distinct spectrum of mutations induced by crocidolite asbestos: clue for 8-hydroxydeoxyguanosine-dependent mutagenesis in vivo. *Cancer Res* 2002;62:99–104.
11. Wisdom R. AP-1: one switch for many signals. *Exp Cell Res* 1999;253:180–185.
12. Ramos-Nino ME, Timblin CR, Mossman BT. Mesothelial cell transformation requires increased AP-1 binding activity and ERK-dependent Fra-1 expression. *Cancer Res* 2002;62:6065–6069.
13. Ni Z, Liu Y, Keshava N, et al. Analysis of K-ras and p53 mutations in mesotheliomas from humans and rats exposed to asbestos. *Mutat Res* 2000;468:87–92.
14. Taniguchi T, Karnan S, Fukui T, et al. Genomic profiling of malignant pleural mesothelioma with array-based comparative genomic hybridization shows frequent non-random chromosomal alteration regions including JUN amplification on 1p32. *Cancer Sci* 2007;98:438–446.
15. Varfolomeev E, Goncharov T, Fedorova AV, et al. c-IAP1 and c-IAP2 are critical mediators of tumor necrosis factor alpha (TNFalpha)-induced NF-kappaB activation. *J Biol Chem* 2008;283: 24295–24299.
16. Gordon GJ, Mani M, Mukhopadhyay L, et al. Expression patterns of inhibitor of apoptosis proteins in malignant pleural mesothelioma. *J Pathol* 2007;211:447–454.
17. Krismann M, Muller KM, Jaworska M, et al. Molecular cytogenetic differences between histological subtypes of malignant mesotheliomas: DNA cytometry and comparative genomic hybridization of 90 cases. *J Pathol* 2002;197:363–371.
18. Sandberg AA, Bridge JA. Updates on the cytogenetics and molecular genetics of bone and soft tissue tumors. Mesothelioma. *Cancer Genet Cytogenet* 2001;127:93–110.
19. Bianchi AB, Mitsunaga SI, Cheng JQ, et al. High frequency of inactivating mutations in the neurofibromatosis type 2 gene (NF2) in primary malignant mesotheliomas. *Proc Natl Acad Sci U S A* 1995;92:10854–10858.
20. Sekido Y, Pass HI, Bader S, et al. Neurofibromatosis type 2 (NF2) gene is somatically mutated in mesothelioma but not in lung cancer. *Cancer Res* 1995;55:1227–12231.
21. Thurneysen C, Opitz I, Kurtz S, et al. Functional inactivation of NF2/merlin in human mesothelioma. *Lung Cancer* 2009;64:140–147.

22. Guled M, Lahti L, Lindholm PM, et al. CDKN2A, NF2, and JUN are dysregulated among other genes by miRNAs in malignant mesothelioma—a miRNA microarray analysis. *Genes Chromosomes Cancer* 2009;48:615–623.
23. Lu W, Lin J, Chen J. Expression of p14ARF overcomes tumor resistance to p53. *Cancer Res* 2002;62:1305–1310.
24. Frizelle SP, Grim J, Zhou J, et al. Re-expression of p16INK4a in mesothelioma cells results in cell cycle arrest, cell death, tumor suppression and tumor regression. *Oncogene* 1998;16:3087–3095.
25. Borczuk AC, Taub RN, Hesdorffer M, et al. P16 loss and mitotic activity predict poor survival in patients with peritoneal malignant mesothelioma. *Clin Cancer Res* 2005;11:3303–3308.
26. Lopez-Rios F, Chuai S, Flores R, et al. Global gene expression profiling of pleural mesotheliomas: overexpression of aurora kinases and P16/CDKN2A deletion as prognostic factors and critical evaluation of microarray-based prognostic prediction. *Cancer Res* 2006;66:2970–2979.
27. Borczuk AC, Cappellini GC, Kim HK, et al. Molecular profiling of malignant peritoneal mesothelioma identifies the ubiquitin-proteasome pathway as a therapeutic target in poor prognosis tumors. *Oncogene* 2007;26:610–617.
28. Yang CT, You L, Yeh CC, et al. Adenovirus-mediated p14(ARF) gene transfer in human mesothelioma cells. *J Natl Cancer Inst* 2000;92:636–641.
29. Altomare DA, Vaslet CA, Skele KL, et al. A mouse model recapitulating molecular features of human mesothelioma. *Cancer Res* 2005;65:8090–8095.
30. Jongsma J, van Montfort E, Vooijs M, et al. A conditional mouse model for malignant mesothelioma. *Cancer Cell* 2008;13:261–271.
31. De Luca A, Baldi A, Esposito V, et al. The retinoblastoma gene family pRb/p105, p107, pRb2/p130 and simian virus-40 large T-antigen in human mesotheliomas. *Nat Med* 1997;3:913–916.
32. Testa JR, Carbone M, Hirvonen A, et al. A multi-institutional study confirms the presence and expression of simian virus 40 in human malignant mesotheliomas. *Cancer Res* 1998;58:4505–4509.
33. Pancaldi C, Balatti V, Guaschino R, et al. Simian virus 40 sequences in blood specimens from healthy individuals of Casale Monferrato, an industrial town with a history of asbestos pollution. *J Infect* 2009;58:53–60.
34. Ziegler A, Seemayer CA, Hinterberger M, et al. Low prevalence of SV40 in Swiss mesothelioma patients after elimination of false-positive PCR results. *Lung Cancer* 2007;57:282–291.
35. Lopez-Rios F, Illei PB, Rusch V, et al. Evidence against a role for SV40 infection in human mesotheliomas and high risk of false-positive PCR results owing to presence of SV40 sequences in common laboratory plasmids. *Lancet* 2004;364:1157–1166.
36. Manfredi JJ, Dong J, Liu WJ, et al. Evidence against a role for SV40 in human mesothelioma. *Cancer Res* 2005;65:2602–2609.
37. Goodman JE, Nascarella MA, Valberg PA. Ionizing radiation: a risk factor for mesothelioma. *Cancer Causes Control* 2009;20:1237–1254.
38. De Bruin ML, Burgers JA, Baas P, et al. Malignant mesothelioma after radiation treatment for Hodgkin lymphoma. *Blood* 2009;113:3679–3681.
39. Carbone M, Emri S, Dogan AU, et al. A mesothelioma epidemic in Cappadocia: scientific developments and unexpected social outcomes. *Nat Rev Cancer* 2007;7:147–154.
40. Karakoca Y, Emri S, Bagci T, et al. Environmentally-induced malignant pleural mesothelioma and HLA distribution in Turkey. *Int J Tuberc Lung Dis* 1998;2:1017–1022.
41. Neri M, Ugolini D, Dianzani I, et al. Genetic susceptibility to malignant pleural mesothelioma and other asbestos-associated diseases. *Mutat Res* 2008;659:126–136.
42. Destro A, Ceresoli GL, Falleni M, et al. EGFR overexpression in malignant pleural mesothelioma. An immunohistochemical and molecular study with clinico-pathological correlations. *Lung Cancer* 2006;51:207–215.
43. Edwards JG, Swinson DE, Jones JL, et al. EGFR expression: associations with outcome and clinicopathological variables in malignant pleural mesothelioma. *Lung Cancer* 2006;54:399–407.
44. Pache JC, Janssen YM, Walsh ES, et al. Increased epidermal growth factor-receptor protein in a human mesothelial cell line in response to long asbestos fibers. *Am J Pathol* 1998;152:333–340.

45. Cortese JF, Gowda AL, Wali A, et al. Common EGFR mutations conferring sensitivity to gefitinib in lung adenocarcinoma are not prevalent in human malignant mesothelioma. *Int J Cancer* 2006;118:521–522.
46. Garland LL, Rankin C, Gandara DR, et al. Phase II study of erlotinib in patients with malignant pleural mesothelioma: a Southwest Oncology Group Study. *J Clin Oncol* 2007;25:2406–2413.
47. Govindan R, Kratzke RA, Herndon JE II, et al. Gefitinib in patients with malignant mesothelioma: a phase II study by the Cancer and Leukemia Group B. *Clin Cancer Res* 2005;11:2300–2304.
48. Foster JM, Gatalica Z, Lilleberg S, et al. Novel and existing mutations in the tyrosine kinase domain of the epidermal growth factor receptor are predictors of optimal resectability in malignant peritoneal mesothelioma. *Ann Surg Oncol* 2009;16:152–158.
49. Hoang CD, Zhang X, Scott PD, et al. Selective activation of insulin receptor substrate-1 and -2 in pleural mesothelioma cells: association with distinct malignant phenotypes. *Cancer Res* 2004;64:7479–7485.
50. Strizzi L, Catalano A, Vianale G, et al. Vascular endothelial growth factor is an autocrine growth factor in human malignant mesothelioma. *J Pathol* 2001;193:468–475.
51. Adachi Y, Aoki C, Yoshio-Hoshino N, et al. Interleukin-6 induces both cell growth and VEGF production in malignant mesotheliomas. *Int J Cancer* 2006;119:1303–1311.

Molecular Prognostic Markers

15

Jason Lester

The development of advanced molecular diagnostic techniques has stimulated interest in identifying potential molecular markers of prognosis in pleural diffuse malignant mesothelioma. Useful prognostic markers not only give valuable information on disease outcome but may provide new therapeutic targets in a disease where established treatments are of limited efficacy. This chapter discusses the molecular markers currently viewed as the most likely candidates to enter clinical practice.

CYCLOOXYGENASE-2

Cyclooxygenase-2 (COX-2) is an enzyme that specifically catalyzes the initial rate-limiting step in the production of prostaglandins. COX-2 plays an important role in solid tumor growth, invasiveness, and angiogenesis, in part through the synthesis of prostaglandins such as prostaglandin E2 (PGE2). In a prospective study, Edwards et al.[1] evaluated COX-2 expression in 48 snap-frozen, surgically resected pleural diffuse malignant mesothelioma tissue specimens using immunohistochemistry and Western blotting. PGE2 was assessed by enzyme immunoassay. High COX-2 expression correlated with poor survival ($p = 0.008$). In multivariate analysis, high COX-2 expression, nonepithelioid cell type, and chest pain were independent predictors of poor prognosis. The presence of PGE2 was demonstrated in all of the samples. The authors concluded that COX-2 expression is a prognostic factor in pleural diffuse malignant mesothelioma and COX-2 is a potential therapeutic target in this disease.

Mineo et al.[2] retrospectively reviewed immunohistochemical expression of COX-2, p21, and p27 divided into high and low expression from histopathologic specimens of 77 consecutive patients. Survival was negatively influenced by high COX-2 expression, low p21 expression, and low p27 expression. COX regression analysis showed that only the combination of high COX-2, low p21, and low p27 expression influenced survival ($p = 0.0001$). The authors suggested that immunohistochemical expression of COX-2, p21, and p27 might be used to guide treatment strategies.

P27

p27 is a cyclin-dependent kinase inhibitor, which binds to cyclin E/cdk2, blocking the G1/S transition step required for cell cycle progression. Beer et al.[3] evaluated the prognostic value of p27 in pleural diffuse malignant mesothelioma by immunohistochemically analyzing tissue samples from 36 patients. The results were quantified by recording the proportion of positively stained nuclei, and these data were tested for association with patient survival. Patients with pleural diffuse malignant mesothelioma showing low p27 expression (<53% of cells positive) had a significantly shorter survival than those with high p27 expression (≥53% of cells positive) ($p = 0.04$). Multivariate analysis showed p27 appeared to be an independent prognostic variable.

Bongiovanni et al.[4] analyzed p27 expression in 27 pleural diffuse malignant mesothelioma (MPM) patients with relatively long-term survival (≥24 months) and a control group of 36 pleural diffuse malignant mesothelioma patients with shorter survival (<24 months). p27 expression was significantly higher in the long-term survival group compared with the shorter survival group (81.41% versus 31.94%; $p < 0.0001$). As might be expected, the epithelioid subtype had a significantly higher p27 expression compared to the biphasic type (59.24% versus 38.94%; $p = 0.02$). Both studies concluded that p27 may be a useful marker to identify pleural diffuse malignant mesothelioma patients with a more favorable prognosis.

P21

Simian virus 40 Large T antigen (SV40 tag) expression has previously been detected in pleural diffuse malignant mesotheliomas.[5,6] The ability of SV40 oncoproteins to inactivate p53 and retinoblastoma tumor suppressor proteins has been proposed as an important step in the pathogenesis of human diffuse malignant mesothelioma.[7] In order to obtain a better understanding of the molecular mechanisms of the pathogenesis of pleural diffuse malignant mesothelioma, Baldi et al.[8] evaluated the expression of the cell cycle inhibitor p21 (a downstream target of p53) in a group of 29 pleural diffuse malignant mesothelioma specimens already characterized for the presence of SV40 tag sequences. p21 expression level was associated with significantly longer median survival ($p < 0.001$). Unlike p27, statistical analysis did not reveal any correlation between p21 expression and histopathologic subtype. The authors concluded that p21 expression has prognostic significance in pleural diffuse malignant mesothelioma and this supported the role of SV40 in the pathogenesis of pleural diffuse malignant mesothelioma.

P16

P16 is a tumor suppressor gene, and as such, p16 gene products have tumor suppressor functions. Dacic et al. carried out a study in 48 pleural diffuse malignant mesothelioma patients to determine the prognostic significance of P16 loss using immunohistochemistry and fluorescence in situ hybridization (FISH).[9] High-density tissue microarrays were constructed from archival formalin-fixed paraffin-embedded samples. Both loss of p16 protein expression by immunohistochemistry and homozygous deletion of P16 by FISH were associated with a worse prognosis. Female gender, positive p16 expression, and lack of P16 deletion significantly predicted longer survival. Statistical analysis showed a very strong correlation between immunohistochemistry and FISH data.

Kobayashi et al.[10] examined p16 expression and P16 gene deletion in specimens from 30 Japanese patients with pleural diffuse malignant mesothelioma using immunohistochemical staining for p16 protein and FISH for the P16 gene. The methylation status of the P16 gene was also examined in 13 patients whose frozen tumor specimens were available using a methylation-specific polymerase chain reaction assay. Among the 30 patients, loss of p16 protein expression was seen in 24 patients (80.0%). Twenty-one patients had homozygous deletions, and nine patients retained the P16 gene. None of the patients with P16 homozygous deletions exhibited p16-positive expression. Three patients who retained the P16 gene did not exhibit p16-positive expression; aberrant P16 methylation was present in two patients with an intact P16 gene but without p16 expression. Patients not expressing p16 had significantly shorter survival than those expressing p16 ($p = 0.04$). Both studies suggest that homozygous deletion of P16 is common in pleural diffuse malignant mesothelioma, leading to loss of p16 protein expression, and that this loss of p16 expression may be associated with a poor prognosis.

GLYCOPROTEIN 90K

90K is a tumor-associated glycoprotein and serum 90K level is reported to indicate a poor prognosis in several cancers. Strizzi et al.[11] used enzyme-linked immunoassay (ELISA) to measure 90K levels in pleural effusions and sera from 28 patients with MPM and 15 patients with benign pleural disease. This was correlated with 90K expression in pleural diffuse malignant mesothelioma and benign pleural disease using immunohistochemistry. The average level of 90K in MPM pleural effusions was significantly higher compared to benign pleural disease. Immunohistochemistry showed expression of 90K in pleural diffuse malignant mesothelioma biopsy sections. A positive correlation between serum 90K levels and pleural diffuse malignant mesothelioma patient survival was seen ($p = 0.006$).

ANGIOGENIC CYTOKINES

Angiogenesis is defined as the induction of blood vessel growth, and it is vital for tumor proliferation. Vascular endothelial growth factor (VEGF), acidic and basic fibroblast growth factors (FGF-1 and FGF-2), and transforming growth factor beta (TGF-beta) are potent angiogenic cytokines. Kumar-Singh et al.[12] reported much higher levels of VEGF, FGF-1 and FGF-2, and TGF-beta in pleural diffuse malignant mesothelioma compared to nonneoplastic mesothelium.[12] High FGF-2 expression was associated with a poorer prognosis. Ohta et al. assessed mRNA expression of VEGF, VEGF type C (VEGF-C), and their receptors together with the microvessel density and microlymphatic vessel density in 54 patients with pleural diffuse malignant mesothelioma.[13] The expression levels of VEGF, VEGF-C, and VEGF receptors were high in all pleural diffuse malignant mesothelioma cell lines. Vessel density was a negative prognostic indicator that correlated with VEGF expression, suggesting both indices could be used as prognostic markers in pleural diffuse malignant mesothelioma.

MIB-1

MIB-1 is a monoclonal antibody, which recognizes the nuclear antigen Ki-67. Ki-67 is a marker of proliferation and has been shown to be prognostic in several tumor types. Beer et al.[14] evaluated MIB-1 as an indicator of prognosis in 41 patients with pleural diffuse malignant mesothelioma. A proliferation index was derived and the results compared with patient survival data. Patients with tumors having a low MIB-1 index lived significantly longer than those with a high MIB-1 index ($p < 0.001$). Comin et al.[15] studied seven long-term survivors with pleural diffuse malignant mesothelioma and a group of control cases with short-term survival. All cases showed MIB-1–positive cells. A statistically significant difference was found in MIB-1 values, with greater proliferation seen in the short-term survival group. It is possible therefore that a proliferation index might be prognostic in pleural diffuse malignant mesothelioma patients.

OSTEOPONTIN

Osteopontin is a glycoprotein involved in cell–matrix interactions. In asbestos-exposed people, high serum levels of osteopontin are correlated with the presence of pleural diffuse malignant mesothelioma but not pleural plaques or interstitial lung disease.[16] In a study by Cappia et al.,[17] 32 long-term survivors (defined as surviving at least 24 months) were matched to 69 short-term survivors (defined as surviving <24 months) using clinical and pathologic features. Immunohistochemical osteopontin expression in pleural diffuse malignant mesothelioma tissue specimens was correlated with survival. Osteopontin expression was significantly lower in long-term compared with short-term survivors, and multivariate analysis showed osteopontin expression to be an independent prognostic factor ($p < 0.0001$).

ESTROGEN RECEPTOR BETA

Female gender is known to be a positive prognostic factor in pleural diffuse malignant mesothelioma. Pinton et al.[18] investigated the role of estrogen receptors (ERs) following this observation. Immunohistochemical analysis revealed intense nuclear ER beta staining in normal pleura that was reduced in tumor tissues. Conversely, neither tumors nor normal pleura stained positive for ER alpha. Multivariate analysis of 78 pleural diffuse malignant mesothelioma patients indicated that ER beta expression is an independent prognostic factor for better survival.

CONCLUSION

Improvements in molecular diagnostic techniques have facilitated the investigation of numerous potential molecular prognostic markers in pleural diffuse malignant mesothelioma. Overexpression of several of these markers has been shown to correlate with outcome; it is likely that several will be integrated into mainstream clinical practice, helping clinicians provide more accurate prognostic information to patients and guiding treatment plans. In addition, the hope is that as more is known about the molecular biology of pleural diffuse malignant mesothelioma, better treatments can be developed, improving the outcome of patients with this devastating disease.

References

1. Edwards JG, Faux SP, Plummer SM, et al. Cyclooxygenase-2 expression is a novel prognostic factor in malignant mesothelioma. *Clin Cancer Res* 2002;8:1857–1862.
2. Mineo TC, Ambrogi V, Cufari ME, et al. May cyclooxygenase-2 (COX-2), p21 and p27 expression affect prognosis and therapeutic strategy of patients with malignant pleural mesothelioma? *Eur J Cardiothorac Surg* 2010;38:245–252.

3. Beer TW, Shepherd P, Pullinger NC. p27 immunostaining is related to prognosis in malignant mesothelioma. *Histopathology* 2001;38:5355–5341.
4. Bongiovanni M, Cassoni P, De Giuli P, et al. p27(kip1) immunoreactivity correlates with long-term survival in pleural malignant mesothelioma. *Cancer* 2001;92:1245–1250.
5. Pepper C, Jasani B, Navabi H, et al. Simian virus 40 large T antigen (SV40LTAg) primer specific DNA amplification in human pleural mesothelioma tissue. *Thorax* 1996;51:1074–1076.
6. Testa JR, Carbone M, Hirvonen A, et al. A multi-institutional study confirms the presence and expression of simian virus 40 in human malignant mesotheliomas. *Cancer Res* 1998;58:4505–4509.
7. Cicala C, Pompetti F, Carbone M. SV40 induces mesotheliomas in hamsters. *Am J Pathol* 1993;142:1524–1533.
8. Baldi A, Groeger AM, Esposito V, et al. Expression of p21 in SV40 large T antigen positive human pleural mesothelioma: relationship with survival. *Thorax* 2002;57:353–356.
9. Dacic S, Kothmaier H, Land S, et al. Prognostic significance of p16/cdkn2a loss in pleural malignant mesotheliomas. *Virchows Arch* 2008;453:627–635.
10. Kobayashi N, Toyooka S, Yanai H, et al. Frequent p16 inactivation by homozygous deletion or methylation is associated with a poor prognosis in Japanese patients with pleural mesothelioma. *Lung Cancer* 2008;62:120–155.
11. Strizzi L, Muraro R, Vianale G, et al. Expression of glycoprotein 90K in human malignant pleural mesothelioma: correlation with patient survival. *J Pathol* 2002;197:218–223.
12. Kumar-Singh S, Weyler J, Martin MJ, et al. Angiogenic cytokines in mesothelioma: a study of VEGF, FGF-1 and -2, and TGF beta expression. *J Pathol* 1999;189:72–78.
13. Ohta Y, Shridhar V, Bright RK, et al. VEGF and VEGF type C play an important role in angiogenesis and lymphangiogenesis in human malignant mesothelioma tumours. *Br J Cancer* 1999; 81:54–61.
14. Beer TW, Buchanan R, Matthews AW, et al. Prognosis in malignant mesothelioma related to MIB 1 proliferation index and histological subtype. *Hum Pathol* 1998;29:246–251.
15. Comin CE, Anichini C, Boddi V, et al. MIB-1 proliferation index correlates with survival in pleural malignant mesothelioma. *Histopathology* 2000;36:26–31.
16. Pass HI, Lott D, Lonardo F, et al. Asbestos exposure, pleural mesothelioma, and serum osteopontin levels. *N Engl J Med* 2005;353:1564–1573.
17. Cappia S, Righi L, Mirabelli D, et al. Prognostic role of osteopontin expression in malignant pleural mesothelioma. *Am J Clin Pathol* 2008;130:58–64.
18. Pinton G, Brunelli E, Murer B, et al. Estrogen receptor-beta affects the prognosis of human malignant mesothelioma. *Cancer Res* 2009;69:4598–4604.

Targeted Gene Therapy 16

Jason Lester

Diffuse malignant mesothelioma is a very aggressive tumor.[1] It is rarely suitable for radical surgery, and other modalities such as radiotherapy and conventional chemotherapy have only modest activity against the neoplasm. For this reason, several novel targeted therapies have been evaluated in an attempt to improve outcomes. As our knowledge has increased regarding the molecular biology of diffuse malignant mesothelioma, the array of potentially useful therapeutic targets has increased. This chapter outlines recent developments in the area of targeted gene therapy and discusses potentially promising future therapeutic approaches for the management of diffuse malignant mesothelioma.

GROWTH FACTORS, THEIR RECEPTORS, AND INHIBITORS

Growth factors and their receptors have already served as ideal targets for novel therapies in various other malignancies. Most have focused on the tyrosine kinase family that controls cell proliferation.

EPIDERMAL GROWTH FACTOR RECEPTOR TYROSINE KINASE INHIBITORS

Epidermal growth factor receptor (EGFR) is overexpressed in a variety of epithelial malignancies. In some lung adenocarcinomas, EGFR gene mutation at the kinase domain predicts response to epidermal growth factor receptor tyrosine kinase inhibitors (EGFR-TKIs). In pleural diffuse malignant mesothelioma, the role of EGFR is less clear and variably reported in the literature.[2,3] The Cancer and Leukemia Group B conducted a phase II study of gefitinib, an oral EGFR-TKI in 43 patients with previously untreated diffuse malignant mesothelioma.[4] Only 2 (4%) patients had a measurable response, and median survival was 6.8 months. EGFR overexpression was seen in almost all patients tested, but gefitinib did not demonstrate any useful activity in diffuse malignant mesothelioma. A similar phase II trial of the EGFR-TKI erlotinib in previously untreated patients with diffuse malignant mesothelioma gave similar results.[5] EGFR was highly expressed in 75% of patient tumors. For 33 patients with measurable disease, there were no objective responses and median overall survival time was 10 months.

Single-agent EGFR-TKIs are not effective in pleural diffuse malignant mesothelioma, despite high expression of EGFR. Activation of the ERK and phosphatidylinositol 3-kinase/Akt downstream pathways is a possible resistance mechanism to EGFR-TKI.

PLATELET-DERIVED GROWTH FACTOR RECEPTOR INHIBITORS

Diffuse malignant mesothelioma cell lines have been found to express platelet-derived growth factor receptor (PDGFR).[6] Imatinib is a selective inhibitor of PDGFR tyrosine kinase. To date, however, imatinib has not demonstrated any useful clinical activity as a monotherapy in diffuse malignant mesothelioma.[7,8] There are preclinical data suggesting a possible synergistic effect of imatinib and chemotherapy, and there are ongoing clinical trials in this area.[9,10]

VASCULAR ENDOTHELIAL GROWTH FACTOR

Among the many factors implicated in angiogenesis, vascular endothelial growth factor (VEGF) has been identified as the most potent and predominant. VEGF is overexpressed in the majority of diffuse malignant mesothelial tumors.[11,12] In addition, VEGF levels are higher in diffuse malignant mesothelioma than in any other solid tumor.[13] Therefore, there is good rationale for investigating VEGF as a potential therapeutic target in diffuse malignant mesothelioma. A variety of antiangiogenic agents have been tried in diffuse malignant mesothelioma, and phase II studies have shown only modest single-agent activity. The CALGB carried out a phase II trial of the PDGFR and VEGFR inhibitor vatalanib in patients with advanced previously untreated pleural diffuse malignant mesothelioma.[14] Forty-seven patients, with a median age of 75 years, were studied. Diffuse malignant mesotheliomas were 77% epithelioid, 9% biphasic, and 10% sarcomatoid. Median overall survival was 10 months. Median progression-free survival was 4.1 months; and the 3-month progression-free survival rate was 55%. No correlation between VEGF and treatment response, progression-free survival, or overall survival was identified, and the authors concluded that vatalanib is ineffective in treating diffuse malignant mesothelioma.[14]

Gemcitabine plus cisplatin is active in diffuse malignant mesothelioma, and Kindler and colleagues added the anti-VEGF antibody bevacizumab to gemcitabine/cisplatin in a multicenter, double-blind, placebo-controlled randomized phase II trial in patients with previously untreated, unresectable diffuse malignant mesothelioma. One hundred eight patients were studied and showed a median progression-free survival time of 6.9 months for the bevacizumab arm and 6.0 months for the placebo arm ($p = 0.88$). The median overall survival times were 15.6 months for the bevacizumab arm and 14.7 months for the placebo arm. Partial response rates were similar between the two arms as well. A higher pretreatment plasma VEGF concentration was associated with shorter progression-free survival and overall survival, independent of the treatment arm. The authors concluded that the addition of the anti-VEGF antibody bevacizumab to the standard gemcitabine/cisplatin treatment regimen does not significantly improve progression-free survival or overall survival in diffuse malignant mesothelioma patients.[15]

A Dutch study treated 40 patients with a confirmed diagnosis of diffuse malignant mesothelioma with increasing doses of thalidomide 100, 200, or maximally 400 mg until progression or unacceptable toxicity.[16] Patients who did not show signs of progression for more than 6 months were considered responders. Forty patients were evaluable for toxicity and efficacy, and 50% had received prior treatment. Eleven patients (27.5%) showed disease stabilization for more than 6 months, and the median survival was 230 days. Most patients were maintained on 200 mg/day as toxicity at this level was minimal.

Karrison et al.[15] have reported on a randomized phase II trial of gemcitabine plus cisplatin with or without the anti-VEGF monoclonal antibody bevacizumab in 108 treatment-naïve patients. Overall, the results were disappointing; there was no significant difference in progression-free survival and median overall survival between the two arms. Bevacizumab-treated patients with low VEGF levels did have significantly longer progression-free survival and median overall survival, suggesting that diffuse malignant mesothelioma tumor profiling may be important in the future for selecting the appropriate treatment for individual patients.

PHOSPHATIDYLINOSITOL 3-KINASE P13K/AKT PATHWAY (mTOR Pathway)

The phosphatidylinositol 3-kinase (PI3K)/AKT pathway, also known as the mTOR (mammalian target of rapamycin) pathway, has been implicated in tumor aggressiveness, in part by mediating cell survival and reducing sensitivity to chemotherapy. Elevated phospho-AKT staining has been observed in human diffuse malignant mesothelioma specimens and in mesothelioma cell xenografts.[17]

When grown as three-dimensional structures, tumor cells can acquire an additional multicellular resistance to apoptosis that may mimic the chemoresistance found in solid tumors. There is evidence that diffuse malignant mesothelioma cell lines, when grown as multicellular spheroids, acquire resistance to a variety of apoptotic stimuli. Inhibitors of the P13K/AKT pathway, particularly rapamycin, have been shown to block much of the acquired resistance of these spheroids, suggesting a positive role for mTOR.[18] In the future, the P13K/AKT pathway may provide a useful therapeutic target for new treatments.

HISTONE DEACETYLASE INHIBITION

Epigenetic regulation of tumor suppressor genes via chromatin condensation and decondensation is being increasingly recognized as having a role in tumorigenesis.[19] Histone acetyltransferases and deacetylases regulate this. Histone deacetylases facilitate chromatin condensation and thereby prevent gene transcription, causing the loss of heterozygosity of tumor suppressors. Inhibition of this process, coupled with a similar inhibition of nonhistone protein deacetylation, ultimately promotes apoptosis, cell cycle arrest, and inhibition of angiogenesis. Histone deacetylase inhibitors inhibit histone deacetylase and other proteins involved in the regulation of gene expression and cell cycle progression. Diffuse malignant mesothelioma expresses the antiapoptotic protein BCL-XL, rendering bcl-xl gene expression a potential therapeutic target. In diffuse malignant mesothelioma cells, histone deacetylase inhibitors induce apoptosis related to the down-regulation of the bcl-xl gene and hence protein expression.[20] Preclinical trials have shown histone deacetylase inhibition to be effective in pleural diffuse malignant mesothelioma cell lines, and in mouse xenograft models, the histone deacetylase inhibitor valproate showed effectiveness in combination with pemetrexed and cisplatin.[21] These preclinical studies have led to a number of early-phase clinical trials in patients with pleural diffuse malignant mesothelioma.[21] In a phase I trial of the histone deacetylase inhibitor vorinostat (suberoylanilide hydroxamic acid) in patients previously treated with chemotherapy, 2 out of 13 patients demonstrated a partial response.[22] Following these results, a multicenter, randomized, placebo-controlled phase III study of the histone deacetylase inhibitor vorinostat in patients with advanced pleural diffuse malignant mesothelioma has been developed and is underway, with the potential for developing a new and effective therapy for these patients.[19]

PROTEASOME INHIBITION

Bortezomib is the first proteasome inhibitor introduced into clinical practice based on significant activity in multiple myeloma. It specifically targets nuclear factor kappa beta (NFκB), blocks the release of key growth factors, has antiangiogenic properties, and is important in apoptosis. In cultured mesothelioma cells, bortezomib increased the cytotoxicity of cisplatin and pemetrexed in a concentration-dependent manner when administered prior to either.[23] Bortezomib may improve outcomes in diffuse malignant mesothelioma patients alone or in combination with standard chemotherapy and is being evaluated in both these settings in clinical trials.

C-Src INHIBITION

The nonreceptor tyrosine kinase c-Src causes changes in proliferation, motility, invasion, survival, and angiogenesis in cancer cells and may be a valid therapeutic target in diffuse malignant mesothelioma. Diffuse malignant mesothelioma cell lines have been shown to express c-Src and demonstrate in vitro sensitivity to the c-Src inhibitor dasatinib.[24] The CALGB is evaluating dasatinib in diffuse malignant mesothelioma patients previously treated with chemotherapy in a phase II trial.

GENE THERAPY

Gene therapy can be defined as the insertion of genes into an individual's cells and tissues to treat a disease. Efficient gene delivery is vital for successful gene therapy, and several vectors have been developed, the commonest and most efficient of which are viral vectors. Viruses replicate by binding to host cells and introducing their genetic material into the replication cycle. The host cell will then carry out the viral genetic instructions and produce additional copies of the virus. Viruses are therefore ideally placed to deliver gene therapy. Put simply, the viral genes that cause disease are removed and replaced by genes encoding the desired effect.

Diffuse malignant mesothelioma is thought to be a good target for gene therapy for several reasons. First, gene therapy is not an effective systemic treatment—it needs to be applied directly to the target tissue; it has not been shown to be effective in malignant diseases that metastasize widely. Diffuse malignant mesothelioma remains localized to the affected hemithorax until relatively late in the disease process. In addition, the pleura can be easily accessed through the chest wall, and the large pleural surface area is ideally suited for rapid gene transfer. Most potential gene therapy strategies have only been tested in the preclinical setting, and relatively few have undergone clinical trials.

SUICIDE GENE THERAPY

Suicide gene therapy involves the transduction of tumor cells with a gene that encodes for specific sensitivity to an exogenous drug, leading to cell death.[25] The herpes simplex virus-1 thymidine kinase suicide gene (HSVtk) makes cells sensitive to ganciclovir, a nucleoside analogue used as an antiviral therapy. In HSVtk-transduced cells, ganciclovir is metabolized to ganciclovir-5′-triphosphate, which results in inhibition of DNA viral replication.[26]

Sterman et al.[27] conducted a phase I dose-escalation clinical trial of adenoviral (Ad)-mediated intrapleural herpes simplex virus thymidine kinase (HSVtk)/ganciclovir gene therapy in 21 previously untreated patients with pleural diffuse malignant mesothelioma. A replication-incompetent recombinant adenoviral vector containing the HSVtk gene was introduced into the pleural cavity of patients followed by 2 weeks of systemic ganciclovir. Dose-limiting toxicity was not reached and the treatment was well tolerated. HSVtk gene transfer was documented in 11 of 20 evaluable patients in a dose-related fashion.

On long-term follow-up, antitumor antibodies and antiadenoviral immune responses were seen. A number of clinical responses were also seen including two long-term survivors.[28] Given the limited amount of gene transfer observed, it was postulated by the authors that Ad.HSVtk may have been effective due to induction of antitumor immune responses—the bystander effect. It is not possible to effect gene transfer to every cancer cell, and the so-called "bystander effect" is increasingly being recognized as an important aspect of tumor cell kill. The bystander effect involves the indirect killing of nontransduced neighboring cells by complex mechanisms, including the induction of a secondary immune response.[29] It is possible, therefore, that systemic augmentation of the immune response to suicide gene therapy with, for example, cytokines, may increase the efficacy of this treatment approach.

CYTOKINE GENE THERAPY

Tumor cells, which express high levels of proinflammatory cytokines, for example, interleukin-2 (IL-2), interferons, and tumor necrosis factor (TNF), will activate the immune system resulting in a more effective antitumor response without having to target specific antigens.[30] Systemic administration of cytokines is associated with significant toxicity, and cytokine gene therapy has the potential to result in high local concentrations of cytokine while limiting more general side effects. Sterman's belief that the majority of cancer cell kill was bystander effect due to secondary antitumor immune responses led them to develop a new vector that would potentially directly induce cell death (like Ad.HSVtk/GCV) and enhance antitumor immune responses by secretion of an immunostimulatory cytokine.

Preclinical studies using an adenoviral vector expressing mouse IFN-β were encouraging enough to justify a phase 1 trial of single-dose intrapleural IFN-β gene transfer using an adenoviral vector (Ad.huIFN-β) in seven patients with pleural diffuse malignant mesothelioma and three patients with metastatic pleural effusions.[31] The treatment was generally well tolerated, and gene transfer was documented in 7 of the 10 patients. Antitumor immune responses were elicited in seven patients, and four patients showed disease stability and/or regression on 18-fluorodeoxyglucose positron emission tomography and computed tomography scans at day 60 after vector infusion.

CONCLUSION

Gene therapy is not yet a therapeutic option for patients with diffuse malignant mesothelioma. The outcomes of phase 1 clinical trials are encouraging and suggest that gene therapy is well tolerated and may have therapeutic benefit. There is a lot of interest in maximizing the bystander effect (leading to indirect tumor cell kill) as gene transfer only transduces a small percentage of tumor cells. Future clinical trials are likely to combine gene therapy with more conventional mesothelioma treatments to reduce tumor volume such as chemotherapy and debulking surgery.

References

1. Cagle PT, Allen TC. Pathology of the pleura: what the pulmonologists need to know. *Respirology* 2011;16:430–438.
2. Okuda K, Sasaki H, Kawano O, et al. Epidermal growth factor receptor gene mutation, amplification and protein expression in malignant pleural mesothelioma. *J Cancer Res Clin Oncol* 2008;134:1105–1111.
3. Destro A, Ceresoli GL, Falleni M, et al. EGFR overexpression in malignant pleural mesothelioma. An immunohistochemical and molecular study with clinico-pathological correlations. *Lung Cancer* 2006;51:207–215.
4. Govindan R, Kratzke RA, Herndon JE II, et al. Gefitinib in patients with malignant mesothelioma: a phase II study by the Cancer and Leukemia Group B. *Clin Cancer Res* 2005;11:2300–2304.
5. Garland LL, Rankin C, Gandara DR, et al. Phase II study of erlotinib in patients with malignant pleural mesothelioma: a Southwest Oncology Group Study. *J Clin Oncol* 2007;25:2406–2413.
6. Langerak AW, De Laat PA, Van Der Linden-Van Beurden CA, et al. Expression of platelet-derived growth factor (PDGF) and PDGF receptors in human malignant mesothelioma in vitro and in vivo. *J Pathol* 1996;178:151–160.
7. Porta C, Mutti L, Tassi G. Negative results of an Italian Group for Mesothelioma (G.I.Me.) pilot study of single-agent imatinib mesylate in malignant pleural mesothelioma. *Cancer Chemother Pharmacol* 2007;59:149–150.
8. Mathy A, Baas P, Dalesio O, et al. Limited efficacy of imatinib mesylate in malignant mesothelioma: a phase II trial. *Lung Cancer* 2005;50:83–86.
9. Bertino P, Porta C, Barbone D, et al. Preliminary data suggestive of a novel translational approach to mesothelioma treatment: imatinib mesylate with gemcitabine or pemetrexed. *Thorax* 2007;62:690–695.
10. Bertino P, Piccardi F, Porta C, et al. Imatinib mesylate enhances therapeutic effects of gemcitabine in human malignant mesothelioma xenografts. *Clin Cancer Res* 2008;14:541–548.
11. Strizzi L, Catalano A, Vianale G, et al. Vascular endothelial growth factor is an autocrine growth factor in human malignant mesothelioma. *J Pathol* 2001;193:468–475.
12. Aoe K, Hiraki A, Tanaka T, et al. Expression of vascular endothelial growth factor in malignant mesothelioma. *Anticancer Res* 2006;26:4833–4836.
13. Linder C, Linder S, Munck-Wikland E, et al. Independent expression of serum vascular endothelial growth factor (VEGF) and basic fibroblast growth factor (bFGF) in patients with carcinoma and sarcoma. *Anticancer Res* 1998;18:2063–2068.
14. Jahan T, Gu L, Kratzke R, et al. Vatalanib in malignant mesothelioma: a phase II trial by the Cancer and Leukemia Group B (CALGB 30107). *Lung Cancer* 2012;76:393–396.
15. Kindler HL, Karrison TG, Gandara DR, et al. Multicenter, double-blind, placebo-controlled, randomized phase II trial of gemcitabine/cisplatin plus bevacizumab or placebo in patients with malignant mesothelioma. *J Clin Oncol* 2012;30:2509–2515.
16. Baas P, Boogerd W, Dalesio O, et al. Thalidomide in patients with malignant pleural mesothelioma. *Lung Cancer* 2005;48:291–296.
17. Altomare DA, You H, Xiao GH, et al. Human and mouse mesotheliomas exhibit elevated AKT/PKB activity, which can be targeted pharmacologically to inhibit tumor cell growth. *Oncogene* 2005;24:6080–6089.
18. Barbone D, Yang TM, Morgan JR, et al. Mammalian target of rapamycin contributes to the acquired apoptotic resistance of human mesothelioma multicellular spheroids. *J Biol Chem* 2008;283:13021–13030.
19. Paik PK, Krug LM. Histone deacetylase inhibitors in malignant pleural mesothelioma: preclinical rationale and clinical trials. *J Thorac Oncol* 2010;5:275–279.

20. Cao XX, Mohuiddin I, Ece F, et al. Histone deacetylase inhibitor downregulation of bcl-xl gene expression leads to apoptotic cell death in mesothelioma. *Am J Respir Cell Mol Biol* 2001;25:562–568.
21. Vandermeers F, Hubert P, Delvenne P, et al. Valproate, in combination with pemetrexed and cisplatin, provides additional efficacy to the treatment of malignant mesothelioma. *Clin Cancer Res* 2009;15:2818–2828.
22. Krug LM, Curley T, Schwartz L, et al. Potential role of histone deacetylase inhibitors in mesothelioma: clinical experience with suberoylanilide hydroxamic acid. *Clin Lung Cancer* 2006;7:257–261.
23. Gordon GJ, Mani M, Maulik G, et al. Preclinical studies of the proteasome inhibitor bortezomib in malignant pleural mesothelioma. *Cancer Chemother Pharmacol* 2008;61:549–558.
24. Tsao AS, He D, Saigal B, et al. Inhibition of c-Src expression and activation in malignant pleural mesothelioma tissues leads to apoptosis, cell cycle arrest, and decreased migration and invasion. *Mol Cancer Ther* 2007;6:1962–1972.
25. Tiberghien P. Use of suicide genes in gene therapy. *J Leuko Biol* 1994;56:203–209.
26. Matthews T, Boehme R. Antiviral activity and mechanism of action of ganciclovir. *Rev Infect Dis* 1988;10(suppl 3):S490–S494.
27. Sterman DH, Treat J, Litzky LA, et al. Adenovirus-mediated herpes simplex virus thymidine kinase/ganciclovir gene therapy in patients with localized malignancy: results of a phase I clinical trial in malignant mesothelioma. *Hum Gene Ther* 1998;9:1083–1092.
28. Sterman DH, Recio A, Vachani A, et al. Long-term follow-up of patients with malignant pleural mesothelioma receiving high-dose adenovirus herpes simplex thymidine kinase/ganciclovir suicide gene therapy. *Clin Cancer Res* 2005;11:7444–7453.
29. Pope IM, Poston GJ, Kinsella AR. The role of the bystander effect in suicide gene therapy. *Eur J Cancer* 1997;33:1005–1016.
30. Vachani A, Moon E, Wakeam E, et al. Gene therapy for mesothelioma and lung cancer. *Am J Respir Cell Mol Biol* 2010;42:385–393.
31. Sterman DH, Recio A, Carroll RG, et al. A phase I clinical trial of single-dose intrapleural IFN-beta gene transfer for malignant pleural mesothelioma and metastatic pleural effusions: high rate of antitumor immune responses. *Clin Cancer Res* 2007;13:4456–4466.

Immunotherapy

17

Jason Lester

Different cancers are considered highly or poorly immunogenic, based on their ability in preclinical models or clinical trials to trigger tumor-specific immune responses. Melanoma is considered strongly immunogenic, followed by renal cancer, while relatively little is known about the ability of diffuse malignant mesothelioma to provoke immune responses. Infiltration of the tumor tissue by high number of $CD8^+$ T cells is associated with lower incidence of lymph node metastasis and longer progression-free survival.[1] This serves as indirect evidence that diffuse malignant mesothelioma is targeted by the immune system. T cells, which infiltrate the tumor tissue, are evidently unable to reject the tumor; however, there is overwhelming evidence that tumor-infiltrating lymphocytes (TILs) can be transformed into robust effector cells by ex vivo manipulation.[2] A clinical trial in melanoma, involving expanding TIL T cells in vitro and injecting them back into lymphodepleted (whole body irradiation with 8 Gy) patients, resulted in >50% objective response rate and some complete responses in advanced multiresistant cases.[2] This autologous system provides strong evidence about the potential of the immune system to eliminate established, bulky tumors but is unlikely to become a mainstream treatment due to individual patient–based complex T-cell culture requirements. An immunologic treatment approach, however, may also work for diffuse malignant mesothelioma, as there are observations that (a) rare spontaneous recovery is associated with improved immune parameters,[3] (b) preclinical models of diffuse malignant mesothelioma respond to immune treatments, and (c) early-phase clinical trials have delivered improved antitumor immune responses and some clinical success. The latter two are discussed in detail below. With increasing knowledge about the immunologic behavior of diffuse malignant mesothelioma and the availability of more effective treatments boosting immune responses, immune therapies supplementing standard treatments will hopefully soon become part of our weaponry against diffuse malignant mesothelioma.

TUMOR-ASSOCIATED ANTIGENS IN DIFFUSE MALIGNANT MESOTHELIOMA

Targeted immunotherapies, apart from those with viral etiology, are based on antigens, which are mutated, expressed uniquely on tumor cells but not on normal cells, or overexpressed on tumor cells. The following tumor-associated antigen (TAA) have been described on diffuse malignant mesothelioma: mesothelin, MUC-1, WT-1, survivin, and 5T4.

MESOTHELIN

Mesothelin is a differentiation antigen, expressed at low levels on normal mesothelial cells lining the pleura, pericardium, and peritoneum. Its expression is highly up-regulated in diffuse malignant mesothelioma and pancreatic cancer and in 50% to 70% of ovarian and lung cancers. The mesothelin gene encodes a precursor protein of 71 kDa that is processed into a 31-kDa and a 40-kDa fragment, the former called megakaryocyte potentiating factor, which is shed, and the latter mesothelin, which is attached to the cell membrane. Cell-bound mesothelin can also shed into the serum. Measuring soluble mesothelin–related proteins has been developed into a mesothelioma test (MESOMARK) and was proposed to be used for diagnostic purposes.[4] Mesothelin is highly expressed on epithelioid but not on the sarcomatoid type of pleural diffuse malignant mesothelioma. The normal function of mesothelin is not known, but cancer-associated mesothelin is able to bind CA125 (MUC16), an ovarian cancer marker, and this may assist intraperitoneal dissemination of ovarian cancer cells. Antimesothelin antibodies have been detected in approximately 40% of cancer patients with mesothelin-expressing tumors, indicating immune engagement and providing the basis to use mesothelin as a therapeutic cancer vaccine.[5] Mesothelin-targeting agents eliciting immune responses are in early-phase clinical trials, such as SS1P and MORAb-009. T-cell epitopes targeting cytotoxic $CD8^+$ T cells against mesothelin-expressing tumors have also been described.[6,7]

SS1P is a recombinant immunotoxin consisting of an antimesothelin antibody linked to a bacterial (Pseudomonas) exotoxin that mediates cell killing by blocking protein synthesis of the cell internalizing and processing it. Phase I studies in diffuse malignant mesothelioma, ovarian cancer, and pancreatic cancer patients concluded that continuous infusion over 10 days is preferable to a 6-dose treatment by prolonging the half-life of the drug and achieving a higher dose. Clinical responses included a partial response, resolution of pleural effusion, and improved quality of life. Further studies, in combination with chemotherapy, are under way.[8]

MORAb-009 is a mouse/human antibody with high affinity for mesothelin, made by Morphotek Inc., a subsidiary of the Eisai Corporation of North America. The mouse sequence contains the recognition sites for mesothelin and is combined with human IgG1 and kappa constant regions. This construct decreases the immunogenicity of the antibody and allows repeated administrations. In vitro, the antibody kills mesothelin-expressing tumor cells via antibody-dependent cellular toxicity. MORAb-009 achieves its pharmacologic effect by two mechanisms, such as by blocking mesothelin's ability to interact with its target and by stimulating the patients' immune system to attack the tumor by specifically destroying those cells bound by MORAb-009. A phase I toxicity study found no limiting toxicity in diffuse malignant mesothelioma, pancreatic cancer, and ovarian cancer patients and found clinical effect in one pancreatic cancer patient.[9]

MUC-1

MUC-1 is an epithelial membrane antigen also present on diffuse malignant mesothelioma cells. It is heavily glycosylated on normal cells, while diffuse malignant mesothelioma cells have an alternatively spliced and differentially glycosylated version from that on normal cells.[10] The expression of the full length MUC-1 gene is >30-fold higher in diffuse malignant mesothelioma than in normal cells.[10] Thus, MUC-1–directed therapies, ongoing in ovarian, breast, and lung cancer, may also be beneficial in patients with diffuse malignant mesothelioma.

WT-1

Wilms tumor 1 protein (WT-1) is a transcription factor expressed in mesodermal tissues during embryogenesis. Its expression is limited in normal tissues, while it is overexpressed in epithelioid diffuse malignant mesothelioma[11] and other solid tumors such as lung, breast, ovarian, and prostate cancer. It serves as a recognition target on diffuse malignant mesothelioma cells for $CD4^+$ and $CD8^+$ T cells generated by analogue peptides in vitro.[12]

SURVIVIN

Survivin is an antiapoptotic protein, preferentially blocking mitochondrial-dependent apoptosis by targeting caspase-8. In healthy tissues, it is important in mitosis, microtubule stability, and embryonic development. While normal, terminally differentiated human cells do not express survivin in general, it is highly expressed in most solid tumors. mRNA and protein levels are significantly elevated in diffuse malignant mesothelioma.[13,14] The accumulation of survivin in diffuse malignant mesothelioma cells is implicated in increased apoptotic defects and resistance to chemotherapy. Survivin is regarded as a prime candidate for immunologic targeting of cancer, as its down-regulation would severely impair the survival capacity of tumor cells. Clinical trials with antisurvivin treatments should certainly consider diffuse malignant mesothelioma as a potential target.

5T4

5T4 is an oncofetal glycoprotein expressed on the cell surface. It has restricted expression in normal tissues but highly overexpressed in numerous malignancies, such as testicular, breast, and colon cancer.[15] Its expression induces multiple changes in cellular dynamics, which collectively induce metastatic disease spread. 5T4 expression is associated with poor disease prognosis in gastric and colorectal carcinomas. Both its expression profile and prognostic value make it an ideal TAA.[16,17] Recent work by Al-Taei demonstrated expression of 5T4 on both epithelioid and sarcomatoid diffuse malignant mesothelioma.[18] In the same study, 5T4-specific T-cell responses were demonstrated in the blood and the pleural effusion of patients with diffuse malignant mesothelioma. 5T4 is currently under development as a target for cancer immunotherapy, for both antibody-based targeted therapy and as a cancer vaccine (TroVax).[19]

COMBINATION CHEMOIMMUNOTHERAPY

The results of using immunotherapy as monotherapy to target bulky, advanced cancers have been largely negative. Future treatments should be designed not only to trigger antitumor immune responses but also to maintain these responses by simultaneously reducing tumor burden and eliminating some of the powerful immunosuppressive effects associated with the tumor. The first step toward this aim is to combine immunotherapy with the standard chemotherapy (pemetrexed and cisplatin) in diffuse malignant mesothelioma, which decreases tumor burden in some patients. The effect of this chemotherapy on immune responses per se has not been studied. Cellular immune responses have been shown to inversely correlate with tumor burden rather than with the administration of chemotherapy in ovarian cancer patients,[20] and although similar studies have not been carried out with pemetrexed, the beneficial immunologic effects of chemotherapy (tumor cell killing, sensitizing tumor cell to immune attack, removing immunosuppressive effects) likely outweigh the direct effect on effector immune cell function.[21] Furthermore, certain types of chemotherapy promote antigen cross-presentation by antigen-presenting cells to prime antitumor CD8$^+$ T-cell responses, generating a "self-vaccinating" effect during chemotherapy.[22] The following immunotherapy approaches in mesothelioma combined with chemotherapy are ongoing or being planned.

MORAb-009

There is an open label clinical trial with MORAb-099, presently recruiting, in diffuse malignant mesothelioma patients receiving standard chemotherapy. Patients receive MORAb-099 in weeks 1 and 2 of every 3-week cycle until disease progression, while pemetrexed and cisplatin are applied on week 1of each cycle for 6 to 12 times. The trial will recruit 16 patients (NCT00923455).

GENE THERAPY WITH TYPE I IFN

Phase I clinical trials, assessing the effects of gene therapy with IFN-β-producing adenovirus (Ad.IFN) administered locally (via pleural catheter), found antitumor immune responses and objective clinical responses in patients treated with a single or two doses, including mixed or partial responses and disease stabilization.[23,24] The Sterman group in Pennsylvania is planning, based on synergistic effects observed in preclinical models, the combination of Ad.IFN with chemotherapy for diffuse malignant mesothelioma patients.[25]

TroVax

TroVax is a cancer vaccine, produced by Oxford BioMedica, that consists of a highly attenuated modified vaccinia virus, strain Ankara, expressing human 5T4. The observation that 5T4 is overexpressed on mesothelial cells[18] is being followed up by a phase I trial in diffuse malignant mesothelioma patients eligible for pemetrexed and cisplatin treatment (Velindre NHS Trust, Cardiff, UK; J. Lester and Z. Tabi).

CYCLOPHOSPHAMIDE TREATMENT TO ELIMINATE REGULATORY T CELLS

The frequency of T regulatory cells is often elevated in the tumor environment hampering effector T-cell function. In a murine mesothelioma model, the effect of gemcitabine combined with a nonspecific immunotherapy was significantly improved when Treg cells were removed.[26] Cyclophosphamide has been shown to have anti-Treg properties in a preclinical model of diffuse malignant mesothelioma.[26] A phase I trial is planned by the team at the National Centre for Asbestos Related Diseases (Perth, Australia) to combine standard chemotherapy with cyclophosphamide treatment.[21]

References

1. Anraku M, Cunningham KS, Yun Z, et al. Impact of tumor-infiltrating T cells on survival in patients with malignant pleural mesothelioma. *J Thorac Cardiovasc Surg* 2008;135:823–829.
2. Rosenberg SA, Restifo NP, Yang JC, et al. Adoptive cell transfer: a clinical path to effective cancer immunotherapy. *Nat Rev Cancer* 2008;8:299–308.
3. Robinson B, Robinson C, Lake R. Localised spontaneous regression in mesothelioma—possible immunological mechanism. *Lung Cancer* 2001;32:197–201.
4. Beyer H, Geschwindt R, Glover C, et al. MESOMARK: a potential test for malignant pleural mesothelioma. *Clin Chem* 2007;53:666–672.
5. Hassan R, Ho M. Mesothelin targeted cancer immunotherapy. *Eur J Cancer* 2008;44:46–53.
6. Yokokawa J, Palena C, Arlen P, et al. Identification of novel human CTL epitopes and their agonist epitopes of mesothelin. *Clin Cancer Res* 2005;11:6342–6351.
7. Thomas AM, Santarsiero LM, Lutz ER, et al. Mesothelin-specific CD8(+) T cell responses provide evidence of in vivo cross-priming by antigen-presenting cells in vaccinated pancreatic cancer patients. *J Exp Med* 2004;200:297–306.
8. Kreitman R, Hassan R, Fitzgerald D, et al. Phase I trial of continuous infusion anti-mesothelin recombinant immunotoxin SS1P. *Clin Cancer Res* 2009;15:5274–5279.
9. Armstrong D, Laheru D, Ma W, et al. A phase 1 study of MORAb-009, a monoclonal antibody against mesothelin in pancreatic cancer, mesothelioma and ovarian adenocarcinoma. *J Clin Oncol, 2007 ASCO Annual Meeting Proceedings Part I* 2007;25 No.:14041.
10. Creaney J, Segal A, Sterrett G, et al. Overexpression and altered glycosylation of MUC1 in malignant mesothelioma. *Br J Cancer* 2008;98:1562–1569.
11. Hecht J, Lee B, Pinkus J, et al. The value of Wilms tumor susceptibility gene 1 in cytologic preparations as a marker for malignant mesothelioma. *Cancer* 2002;96:105–109.
12. May R, Dao T, Pinilla-Ibarz J, et al. Peptide epitopes from the Wilms' tumor 1 oncoprotein stimulate CD4+ and CD8+ T cells that recognize and kill human malignant mesothelioma tumor cells. *Clin Cancer Res* 2007;13:4547–4555.
13. Falleni M, Pellegrini C, Marchetti A, et al. Quantitative evaluation of the apoptosis regulating genes Survivin, Bcl-2 and Bax in inflammatory and malignant pleural lesions. *Lung Cancer* 2005;48:211–216.
14. Zaffaroni N, Costa A, Pennati M, et al. Survivin is highly expressed and promotes cell survival in malignant peritoneal mesothelioma. *Cell Oncol* 2007;29:453–466.
15. Hole N, Stern P. A 72 kD trophoblast glycoprotein defined by a monoclonal antibody. *Br J Cancer* 1988;57:239–246.
16. Amato R. 5T4-modified vaccinia Ankara: progress in tumor-associated antigen-based immunotherapy. *Expert Opin Biol Ther* 2010;10:281–287.
17. Amato R. 5T4-modified vaccinia ankara: progress in tumor-associated antigen-based immunotherapy. *Expert Opin Biol Ther* 2007;7:1463–1469.
18. Al-Taei S, Salimu J, Lester JF, et al. Overexpression and potential targeting of the oncofoetal antigen 5T4 in malignant pleural mesothelioma. *Lung Cancer* 2012;77:312–318.
19. Elkord E, Shablak A, Stern P, et al. 5T4 as a target for immunotherapy in renal cell carcinoma. *Expert Rev Anticancer Ther* 2009;9:1705–1709.
20. Coleman S, Clayton A, Mason MD, et al. Recovery of CD8+ T-cell function during systemic chemotherapy in advanced ovarian cancer. *Cancer Res* 2005;65:7000–7006.

21. McCoy M, Nowak A, Lake R. Chemoimmunotherapy: an emerging strategy for the treatment of malignant mesothelioma. *Tissue Antigens* 2009;74:1–10.
22. Obeid M, Tesniere A, Ghiringhelli F, et al. Calreticulin exposure dictates the immunogenicity of cancer cell death. *Nat Med* 2007;13:54–61.
23. Sterman D, Recio A, Carroll R, et al. A phase I clinical trial of single-dose intrapleural IFN-beta gene transfer for malignant pleural mesothelioma and metastatic pleural effusions: high rate of antitumor immune responses. *Clin Cancer Res* 2007;13:4456–4466.
24. Sterman D, Recio A, Haas A, et al. A phase I trial of repeated intrapleural adenoviral-mediated interferon-beta gene transfer for mesothelioma and metastatic pleural effusions. *Mol Ther* 2010;18:852–860.
25. Vachani A, Moon E, Wakeam E, et al. Gene therapy for mesothelioma and lung cancer. *Am J Respir Cell Mol Biol* 2010;42:385–393.
26. van der Most R, Currie A, Mahendran S, et al. Tumor eradication after cyclophosphamide depends on concurrent depletion of regulatory T cells: a role for cycling TNFR2-expressing effector-suppressor T cells in limiting effective chemotherapy. *Cancer Immunol Immunother* 2009;58:1219–1228.

Molecular Diagnostics

18

Richard L. Attanoos

Molecular analytic techniques have established a pivotal role in the diagnosis of a wide variety of soft tissue tumors. This is because most malignant soft tissue tumors have clonal chromosomal abnormalities that are entity specific. To date, no complementary analysis (histochemistry, immunohistochemistry, and electron microscopic studies) to morphology allows for 100% definitive diagnosis of diffuse malignant mesothelioma. This has prompted researchers to seek out specific diagnostic and prognostic molecular markers in diffuse malignant mesothelioma. Moreover, the identification of a specific molecular marker may serve as a determinant of a premalignant state or identify those cases associated with asbestos. The former would have potential clinical implications for health care surveillance, the latter potential legal implications. This chapter discusses the role of molecular diagnostics in the identification of diffuse malignant mesothelioma and its mimics. The role of prognostic markers in diffuse malignant mesothelioma and mechanisms of asbestos-mediated tumorigenesis are covered in other chapters.

Diffuse malignant mesothelioma has the capacity to mimic a wide variety of histogenetically distinct tumors and reactive conditions. Because the entire morphologic spectrum of diffuse malignant mesothelioma encompasses such a wide differential diagnostic list of conditions, there is a necessary focus on the common diagnostic dilemmas and most useful areas where molecular analysis has a role in diagnosis.

DIFFUSE MALIGNANT MESOTHELIOMA

Various analytic techniques have been used to study the molecular biology of diffuse malignant mesothelioma.[1,2] Clonal karyotypic alterations have been reported as common in diffuse malignant mesothelioma, and most of these cases have shown multiple chromosomal abnormalities involving chromosomes 1, 3, 6, 9, and 22.[3–8] Chromosomal deletions are more common than gains. These molecular changes have been reported in epithelioid, biphasic, and sarcomatoid subtypes of the tumor and in pleural and peritoneal cases. Single cytogenetic change in diffuse malignant mesothelioma is very uncommon. The most common cytogenetic abnormality in diffuse malignant mesothelioma is a deletion in 9p21, the locus of CDKN2A ($p16^{INK4a}$), and CDKN2B ($p15^{INK4b}$). A CDKN2A deletion is also an adverse prognostic factor in diffuse malignant mesothelioma. These tumor suppressor genes encode for cyclin-dependent kinase inhibitor proteins, which mediate the retinoblastoma pathway and regulate the cell cycle during the G1/S phase. Without the inhibition of CDK4 kinase activity, cells are able to lose their cell cycle control and undergo neoplastic transformation.

Comparative genomic hybridization (CGH) focuses on measuring DNA chromosomal imbalances. No specific chromosome anomaly has been found to characterize diffuse malignant mesothelioma. While a number of recurrent abnormalities have been found, interlaboratory variations exist casting doubt on the consistency of results. The more recurrent anomalies found by different investigators in diffuse malignant mesothelioma include monosomy of chromosomes 4 and 22; polysomy of chromosomes 5, 7, and 20; and loss at 1p21–p22, 3p21, 6q15–q21, 9p21–p22, and 22q12. None of these abnormalities is specific for diffuse malignant mesothelioma.

Loss of heterozygosity (LOH) studies that have located possible tumor suppressor genes at 1p, 3p, and 9p have indicated the complex nature of chromosomal imbalances in diffuse malignant mesothelioma.[8] The CDKN2A gene has been found to be homozygously deleted in a large number of diffuse malignant mesotheliomas.

Fluorescence in situ hybridization studies using formalin-fixed paraffin-embedded cases of pleural diffuse malignant mesothelioma and incorporating centromeric probes found infrequent chromosome loss and frequent added chromosomes especially in chromosomes 1, 3, 6, 7, 11, and 17. No specificity was found for these changes.[9]

There is no consistent correlation between subtype (epithelioid, sarcomatous, or biphasic) based on molecular cytogenetic, fluorescent in situ hybridization, CGH, or other analytic techniques. The cytogenetic studies have underlined the complexity and heterogeneity of chromosomal abnormalities in diffuse malignant mesothelioma. This supports the view that diffuse malignant mesothelioma results from the cumulative effect of a number of acquired genetic events, which lead to inactivation of multiple tumor suppressor genes in a multistep process.

DIFFUSE MALIGNANT MESOTHELIOMA VERSUS LUNG CARCINOMA

In the pleura, a common problem is to distinguish epithelioid diffuse malignant mesothelioma from lung carcinoma, mainly adenocarcinoma. Immunohistochemistry is effective in distinguishing between the two tumors. CGH has also been used as a potential diagnostic tool. Bjorkqvist et al.[9] found that unlike diffuse malignant mesothelioma (where losses in 4q, 6q, and 14q were most common), gains predominated over losses in lung cancer especially at 1q, 5p, 6p, 7p, and 8q. Despite the significant difference in frequency of gains and losses, the authors concluded that that CGH cannot be used as a definitive discriminatory method in distinguishing non–small cell lung carcinoma and diffuse malignant mesothelioma.[10,11,12]

Deletions and rearrangements of 3p (particularly 3p21) have been reported in a high percentage of diffuse malignant mesotheliomas. Such deletions have also been reported in a number of other tumors (small and non–small cell lung cancers, renal cell carcinoma, breast cancer, ovarian cancer, and lymphoma), and hence, it has been suggested that loss of 3p may represent an important generalized tumorigenic event common to various cancers. Many of these cancers morphologically mimic diffuse malignant mesothelioma.

It has been reported that gains in X, 1p, 10q, and 18q and high level amplification in 8q are seen only in adenocarcinoma, whereas losses in 10q and 18q occurred only in diffuse malignant mesothelioma. The potential utility of this in a diagnostic setting has been raised but requires validation.

Apoptosis and expression of apoptosis-regulating proteins (*bcl-2*, *mcl-1*, *bcl-X*, and *bax*) were studied in histologic sections of 35 cases of diffuse malignant mesothelioma and 21 cases of metastatic lung adenocarcinoma.[2] The results show that *bcl-X*, *mcl-1*, and *bax* are abundantly expressed in diffuse malignant mesothelioma, mesothelioma cell lines, and nonneoplastic mesothelial cells. When expressed, *bcl-2* inhibits apoptosis, as shown by a significantly lower level of apoptosis in *bcl-2*–positive diffuse malignant mesothelioma compared with other tumors.[2] The differentiation of diffuse malignant mesothelioma from lung cancers, particularly adenocarcinoma, has shown that no molecular marker is specific to allow absolute differentiation of these tumors.

REACTIVE VERSUS NEOPLASTIC MESOTHELIAL PROLIFERATIONS

Differentiating reactive mesothelial proliferations from diffuse malignant mesothelioma is particularly challenging, particularly in small biopsy specimens. If a serosal biopsy fails to demonstrate frank invasion, then there is no definitive diagnosis of diffuse malignant mesothelioma. Indeed, there exists no cytomorphologic features or immunohistochemical marker, which is 100% specific or sensitive for diffuse malignant mesothelioma. Immunohistochemical markers can readily identify cells of mesothelial origin. The role of epithelial membrane antigen, p53, desmin, GLUT-1, P-glycoprotein, and platelet-derived growth factor receptor β-chain is discussed in other chapters. The first four markers appear most useful, but there exist interpretive pitfalls.

Molecular analysis has emerged as potentially useful in this diagnostic setting. Deletion involving the 9p21 locus, the site of the cyclin-dependent kinase inhibitor 2A/p16 gene (*p16/CDKN2A*), frequently occurs in diffuse malignant mesothelioma.[13] Homozygous deletion has been reported in 22% to 74% of diffuse malignant mesotheliomas. It has been proposed that FISH on paraffin-embedded sections for *p16/CDKN2A* deletion can be a clinically useful marker to confirm a diagnosis of malignancy, particularly in biopsies with limited material that lack definitive evidence of invasion. Moreover, 9p21 locus deletion by FISH on cytologic preparations and tissue sections has been reported and suggested as a clinical assay for diagnosing diffuse malignant mesothelioma. Illei et al.[14] identified homozygous *p16/CDKN2A* deletion in 85.7% (6/7) of cases with malignant cytology and 100% (6/6) with suspicious cytology; no deletion was detected in 19 cytologically negative specimens.

The possible use of telomerase reverse transcriptase to differentiate diffuse malignant mesothelioma from reactive mesothelial hyperplasia has been described although results require validation.[15]

DIFFUSE MALIGNANT MESOTHELIOMA VERSUS SYNOVIAL SARCOMA

There is an increasing awareness of the diagnostic dilemmas that exist in distinguishing sarcomatoid diffuse malignant mesothelioma from synovial sarcoma. Synovial sarcoma is an aggressive tumor that frequently (in 90% of the cases) arises in the limbs of young adults. However, it may arise at other locations in the body, including heart, abdominal wall, mediastinum, and lung. There is a male predilection. Synovial sarcoma may arise in the pleura, pericardium, or peritoneum. Diffuse malignant mesotheliomas may show an epithelioid, biphasic, or sarcomatoid morphology; and synovial sarcoma also has a varied appearance with monophasic and biphasic forms or spindle cell, biphasic, epithelioid, and poorly differentiated variants.[16] Synovial sarcoma may also mimic fibrosarcoma, solitary fibrous tumor, leiomyosarcoma, and malignant peripheral nerve sheath tumors. All except solitary fibrous tumor rarely arise in the serosa. There exist subtle morphologic features seen in synovial sarcoma that are infrequent in diffuse malignant mesothelioma, such as the hemangiopericytomatous cell distribution and calcification, but none is specific.

Immunohistochemistry plays a limited role, with no marker specific for either entity. Importantly, the mesothelial marker calretinin may be positive in synovial sarcoma, and there may be focal cytokeratin and vimentin positivity. WT-1 (as a mesothelial marker, negative in synovial sarcoma) and bcl-2, CD 56, and CD 99 (positive in synovial sarcoma) may be useful to favor synovial sarcoma over diffuse malignant mesothelioma.

Molecular diagnostic studies have been regarded as a definitive means of identifying synovial sarcoma. The specific translocation t(X;18)(p11.2;q11.2) leads to the formation of a fusion gene between SSXT (also termed SYT) on chromosome 18 and one of two adjacent genes, SSX1 or SSX2. The fusion product encodes a nuclear protein effecting gene expression. This translocation is present in both monophasic and biphasic variants. The translocation is present in more than 90% of synovial sarcomas and in about 30% is the sole cytogenetic anomaly. The demonstration of the t(X;18) can be accomplished by cytogenetics or multifluor/spectral karyotypic analysis (SKY) (on fresh tissue), by fluorescent in situ hybridization (on fresh, fixed, or paraffin-embedded tissue), or by reverse transcriptase polymerase chain reaction (RT-PCR) (on fresh or paraffin-embedded tissue)[17] (Fig. 18-1). The latter technique affords the ability of detecting the fusion products and correlating

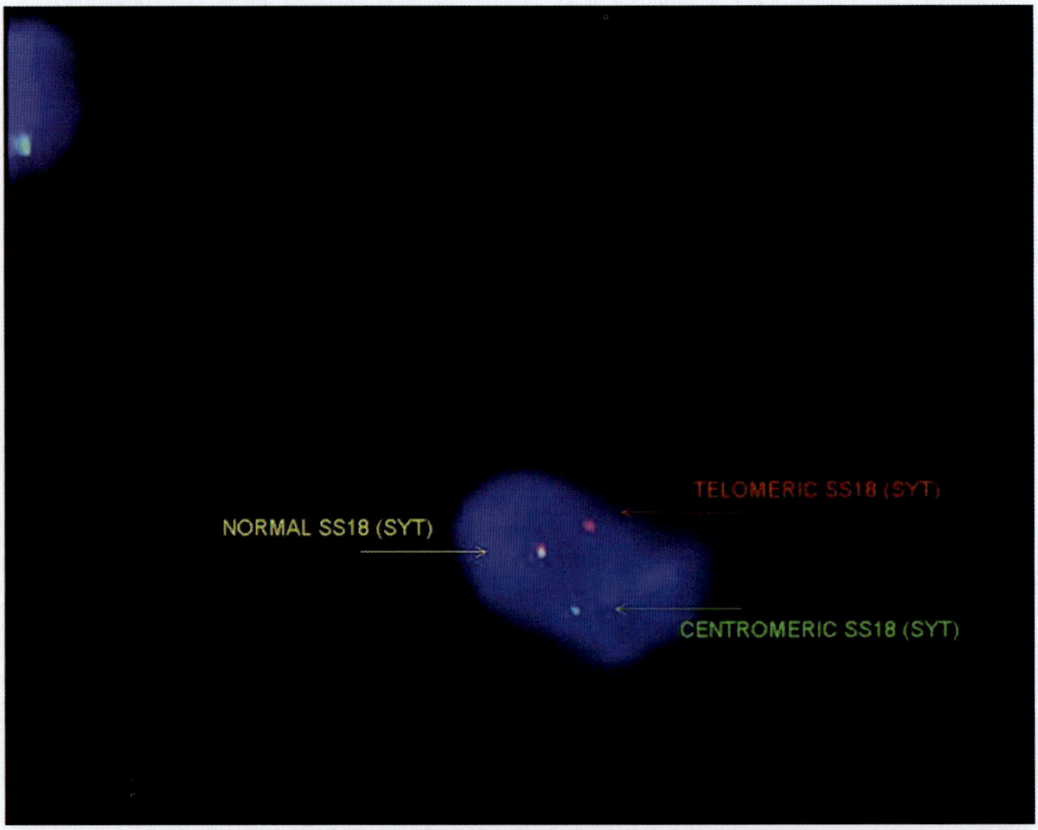

FIGURE 18-1: Fluorescent in situ hybridization of synovial sarcoma using commercial break apart probes to X: 18 demonstrate the translocation within tumor cells.

histologic type and translocation. The SSXT-SSX1 is associated with high proliferative activity, adverse prognosis,[18] and biphasic subtype, and SSXT-SSX2 fusion product with monophasic morphology.[19]

DIFFUSE MALIGNANT MESOTHELIOMA VERSUS DESMOPLASTIC SMALL ROUND-CELL TUMOR

Desmoplastic small round cell tumor (DSRCT) is a rare soft tissue tumor with diverse morphologic and immunophenotypic characteristics arising from putative uncommitted mesenchymal stem cells. The pathologic and clinical aspects of the tumor were first delineated by Gerald and Rosai.[20,21] This uncommon tumor is characterized by small, poorly differentiated cells separated by a prominent desmoplastic stroma and multilineage differentiation. The immunohistochemical profile is characterized by the coexpression of epithelial (keratin and epithelial membrane antigen), mesenchymal (vimentin and desmin, but not actin), and occasionally neural (neuron-specific enolase) antigens.[22] The most common primary sites for DSRCT relate to the serosal lining of body cavities, namely, the pleura, peritoneum, and paratesticular region. DSRCT has a strong correlation with the specific genetic translocation t(11;22)(p13;q12).[23,24] This translocation fuses the Ewing sarcoma gene EWS on chromosome 22 with the Wilms tumor gene WT-1 on chromosome 11.

DIFFUSE MALIGNANT MESOTHELIOMA AND PRIMITIVE NEUROECTODERMAL TUMORS

Most (80%) Ewing sarcomas and various primitive neuroectodermal tumors like the pleuropulmonary Askin tumor contain the characteristic translocation between the long arms of chromosomes 11 and 22; t(11;22) (q24;q12).[25] The chromosome 11 Friend leukemia integration 1 (FLI 1) gene is a transcription factor, and fusion with chromosome 22 EWS is oncogenic. The same translocation has been reported in other small round cell tumors such as olfactory neuroblastoma, small cell osteosarcoma, and mesenchymal chondrosarcoma. These are all exceptional in the differential diagnosis with diffuse malignant mesothelioma.

FLI-1 protein is detectable by immunohistochemistry and commonly incorporated in the differential diagnosis of small round cell tumors as a more specific but less sensitive marker than CD 99. FLI-1 nuclear expression is seen in various endothelial tumors, Merkel cell carcinoma, Ewing sarcoma, lymphoblastic leukemia, and a subpopulation of normal lymphocytes.

DIFFUSE MALIGNANT MESOTHELIOMA VERSUS CLEAR CELL SARCOMA (MELANOMA OF SOFT PARTS)

Pseudomesotheliomatous clear cell sarcoma of the pleura has been reported.[26] The use of cytogenetic analysis allowed for the distinction of the tumor from other considered diagnoses. Clear cell sarcoma has a translocation of t(12;22) (q13;q12) in approximately 75% cases, which is not present in cutaneous melanoma cases.[27] This t(12;22) translocation fuses the ATF gene, which encodes a transcription factor (on chromosome 12) with the EWS gene (on chromosome 22). The translocation may be detected by karyotyping or in situ hybridization. The fusion product ATF-1-EWS is detectable by RT-PCR. This translocation has not been reported in diffuse malignant mesothelioma.

SUMMARY

Molecular diagnostics has an important role in the diagnosis of a variety of soft tissue tumors and hematologic malignancies. The absence of a specific chromosomal change in diffuse malignant mesothelioma is unfortunate, since such a finding would assist in the diagnosis of diffuse malignant mesothelioma, particularly in problematic cases. To date, the most useful role of molecular analysis is in the confirmation of other tumors that mimic diffuse malignant mesothelioma, including synovial sarcoma and DSRCT, both of which may be serosal tumors and mimic diffuse malignant mesothelioma, and both may have overlapping immunophenotypic profiles with mesothelioma. Both have distinctive molecular translocations, which have not been reported in diffuse malignant mesothelioma. The exciting potential role of using molecular biomarkers for the early detection of malignant mesothelial proliferations in cytology and small biopsy specimens appears to be the most likely direct value of this technology for positive diffuse malignant mesothelioma diagnosis.

References

1. Lee W-C, Testa JR. Somatic genetic alterations in human malignant mesothelioma (review). *Int J Oncol* 1999;14:181–188.
2. Sandberg AA, Bridge JA. Updates on the cytogenetics and molecular genetics of bone and soft tissue tumors. Mesothelioma. *Cancer Genet Cytogenet* 2001;127:93–110.
3. Gibas Z, Li FP, Antman KH, et al. Chromosome changes in malignant mesothelioma. *Cancer Genet Cytogenet* 1986;20:191–201.
4. Krismann M, Muller KM, Jaworska M, et al. Molecular cytogenetic differences between histological subtypes of malignant mesotheliomas: DNA cytometry and comparative genomic hybridization of 90 cases. *J Pathol* 2002;197:363–371.
5. Bell DW, Jhanwar SC, Testa JR. Multiple regions of allelic loss from chromosome arm 6q in malignant mesothelioma. *Cancer Res* 1997;57:4057–4062.
6. Knuutila S, Tammilehto L, Mattson K. Chromosomal abnormalities in human malignant mesothelioma. In: Jaurand M-C, Bigner J, eds. *The Mesothelial Cell and Mesothelioma*. New York, NY: Marcel Dekker, Inc.; 1994:245–252.
7. Taguchi T, Jhanwar SC, Siegfried JM, et al. Recurrent deletions of specific chromosomal sites in 1p, 3p, 6q, and 9p in human malignant mesothelioma. *Cancer Res* 1993;53:4349–4355.
8. Lee WC, Balsara B, Liu, Z, et al. Loss of heterozygosity analysis defines a critical region in chromosome 1p22 commonly deleted in human malignant mesothelioma. *Cancer Res* 1996;56: 4297–4301.
9. Björkqvist A-M, Tammilehto L, Nordling S, et al. Mesothelioma and lung carcinomas. *Cancer Genet Cytogenet* 1997;98:149.
10. Segers K, Ramael M, Singh SK, et al. Detection of numerical chromosomal aberrations in paraffin embedded malignant pleural mesothelioma by non-isotopic *in situ* hybridization. *J Pathol* 1995;175:219–226.
11. Kobashi Y, Matsushima T, Irei T. Clinicopathological analysis of lung cancer resembling malignant pleural mesothelioma. *Respirology* 2005;10:660–665.

12. Shivapurkar N, Virmani AK, Wistuba II, et al. Deletions of chromosome 4 at multiple sites are frequent in malignant mesothelioma and small cell lung carcinoma. *Clin Cancer Res* 1999;5:17–23.
13. Cheng JQ, Jhanwar SC, Klein WM, et al. p16 alterations and deletion mapping of 9p21-p22 in malignant mesothelioma. *Cancer Res* 1994;54:5547–5551.
14. Illei PB, Ladanyi M, Rusch VW, et al. The use of CDKN2A deletion as a diagnostic marker for malignant mesothelioma in body cavity effusions. *Cancer* 2003;99:51–56.
15. Kamaki F, Kawai T, Churg A, et al. Expression of telomerase reverse transcriptase (TERT) in malignant mesothelioma. *Mod Pathol* 2001;14:222A.
16. Fisher C. Synovial sarcoma. *Curr Diagn Pathol* 1994;1:13–18.
17. Turc-Carel C, Dal Cin P, Limon J, et al. Translocation X;18 in synovial sarcoma. *Cancer Genet Cytogenet* 1986;23:93.
18. Inagaki H, Nagasaka T, Otsuka T, et al. Association with SYT—SSX fusion types with proliferative activity and prognosis in synovial sarcoma. *Mod Pathol* 2000;13:482.
19. Kawai A, Woodruff J, Healey JH, et al. SSX—SYT gene fusion as a determinant of morphology and prognosis in synovial sarcoma. *N Engl J Med* 1998;338:153.
20. Gerald WL, Rosai J. Desmoplastic small cell tumor with divergent differentiation. *Pediatr Pathol* 1989;9:177–183.
21. Gerald WL, Ladanyi M, de Alava E, et al. Clinical, pathologic, and molecular spectrum of tumors associated with t(11;22)(p13;q12): desmoplastic small round-cell tumor and its variants. *J Clin Oncol* 1998;16:3028–3036.
22. Ordóñez NG. Desmoplastic small round cell tumor. I: a histopathologic study of 39 cases with emphasis on unusual histological patterns. *Am J Surg Pathol* 1998;22:1303–1313.
23. Gerald WL, Ladanyi M, de Alava E, et al. Desmoplastic small round-cell tumor: a recently recognized tumor type associated with a unique gene fusion. *Adv Anatomic Pathol* 1995;2:341–345.
24. Ladanyi M, Gerald WL. Specificity of the EWS/WT1 gene fusion for desmoplastic small round cell tumour. *J Pathology* 1996;180:462.
25. Turc-Carel C, Aurias A, Mugneret F, et al. Chromosomes in Ewings' sarcoma an evaluation of 85 cases of remarkable consistency of t(11;22)(q24; q12). *Cancer Genet Cytogenet* 1988;32:229.
26. Joshi A, McAndrew N, Birdsall S, et al. Clear cell sarcoma mimicking malignant pleural mesothelioma. *Histopathology* 2008;53:359–361.
27. Bridge JA, Borek DA, Neff JR, et al. Chromosomal abnormalities in clear cell sarcoma: implications for histogenesis. *Am J Clin Pathol* 1990;93:26.

Cancer Stem Cells

19

Timothy Craig Allen

Cancer stem cell theory has been unequivocally accepted for a decade.[1] Originally identified in neoplasms of the hematopoietic system, cancer stem cells have also been extensively studied in solid tumors.[1–4] Stem cells' most important property is self-renewal. Cancer stem cells are a rare population of stem cells that drive tumorigenesis by their infinite potential for self-renewal.[1] There are several cell surface antigenic markers that are now considered common in stem cells in several solid tumors, including CD9, CD24, CD26, CD44, CD90, CD133, SP, Bmi-1, uPAR, and ABCG2.[2,3,5–7]

Cacciotti et al.[8] proposed that Akt activation induces cell survival of a subpopulation of transformed stem cells and that Akt signaling may be a therapeutic target to overcome resistance to conventional therapies. Lau and Kane[9] found that stem cells are recruited to malignant mesothelioma spheroids and that the chemokine SDF1 recruits stem cells and is a potential target for therapy.

It is thought that cancer stem cells persist in tumors and cause tumor relapse after chemotherapy and that these cells are responsible for tumor resistance and recurrence.[6] Cortes-Dericks and colleagues showed the expression of cancer stem cell markers CD133, Bmi-1, uPAR, and ABCG2 in both normal mesothelial cells and cells from a pleural diffuse malignant mesothelioma cell line. Cells positive with Bmi-1, uPAR, and ABCG2 conferred chemoresistance to cisplatin and pemetrexed, a common treatment regimen used in patients with diffuse malignant mesothelioma. Normal mesothelial cells showed no chemoresistance properties. CD133-positive cells showed chemoresistance properties in both normal cells and mesothelial cell line cells. That cancer stem cells may impart drug resistance to cisplatin and pemetrexed in cells from diffuse malignant mesothelioma cell lines suggests that targeting these drug-resistant cells may provide more focused and effective chemotherapeutic regimens for pleural diffuse malignant mesothelioma.

Ghani et al.[7] found that CD26 expression closely correlates with CD24 in sarcomatoid diffuse malignant mesothelioma cell lines and that CD9- and CD24-positive cells had a higher potential to generate spheroid colonies than did stem cells negative for CD9 and CD24. The CD9- and CD24-positive stem cells also tended to generate larger tumors in a mouse transplantation assay.

A recent study by Yamazaki et al.[10] examining cancer stem cell markers found that CD44 was expressed homogeneously in all cell lines, CD24 is the primary stem cell marker in many diffuse malignant mesotheliomas, and CD26, highly expressed in most diffuse malignant mesothelioma patient specimens, is associated with immune regulation and signal transduction. The authors also found that CD24 correlates with drug resistance and proliferation potentials and CD26 correlates with asymmetric cell division and invasion potentials. Further, signals downstream from these markers may be targets for cancer stem cell–oriented therapies. Up-regulation of cancer-related genes such as IGFBP3 and IGFBP7 has been shown to be correlated with CD24, CD26, or both. IGFBP7 is reportedly involved in ERK phosphorylation, which is a key step in the development of diffuse malignant mesothelioma by asbestos exposure.

Expression patterns of CD24 and CD26 differ depending on diffuse malignant mesothelioma cell types; and cancer stem cell signatures and ERK signaling pathways also differ depending on cancer stem cell marker expressions.[10] These cancer stem cell markers are therefore potential targets for cancer stem cell–oriented diffuse malignant mesothelioma therapies. As such, their relative expression patterns, both separately and in combination, may be important.[10] Future studies will likely further elucidate the role of cancer stem cells in the diagnosis, prognosis, and treatment of diffuse malignant mesothelioma.

References

1. Reya T, Morrison SJ, Clarke MF, et al. Stem cells, cancer, and cancer stem cells. *Nature* 2001; 414:105–111.
2. Li C, Heidt DG, Dalerba P, et al. Identification of pancreatic cancer stem cells. *Cancer Res* 2007; 67:1030–1037.
3. Gao MQ, Choi YP, Kang S, et al. CD24+ cells from hierarchically organized ovarian cancer are enriched in cancer stem cells. *Oncogene* 2010;29:2672–2680.
4. Frank NY, Schatton T, Frank MH. The therapeutic promise of the cancer stem cell concept. *J Clin Invest* 2010;120:41–50.
5. Visvader JE, Lindeman GJ. Cancer stem cells in solid tumours: accumulating evidence and unresolved questions. *Nat Rev Cancer* 2008;8:755–768.
6. Cortes-Dericks L, Carboni GL, Schmid RA, et al. Putative cancer stem cells in malignant pleural mesothelioma show resistance to cisplatin and pemetrexed. *Int J Oncol* 2010;37:437–444.
7. Ghani FI, Yamazaki H, Iwata S, et al. Identification of cancer stem cell markers in human malignant mesothelioma cells. *Biochem Biophys Res Commun* 2011;404:735–742.
8. Cacciotti P, Barbone D, Porta C, et al. SV40-dependent AKT activity drives mesothelial cell transformation after asbestos exposure. *Cancer Res* 2005;65:5256–5262.
9. Lau BW, Kane AB. SDF1/CXCL12 is involved in recruitment of stem-like progenitor cells to orthotopic murine malignant mesothelioma spheroids. *Anticancer Res* 2010;30:2153–2160.
10. Yamazaki H, Naito M, Ghani FI, et al. Characterization of cancer stem cell properties of CD24 and CD26-positive human malignant mesothelioma cells. *Biochem Biophys Res Commun* 2012;419: 529–536.

Index

Note: Page numbers in *italics* indicates figures and those followed by t indicates tables